VIVA IN BIOCHEMISTRY

(How much relevant to speak and in which style?)

Other Books by Dr. S.P. Singh

- Textbook of Biochemistry, 6/e
- Practical Manual of Biochemistry, 8/e
- A Textbook of Dental Biochemistry, 3/e
- Concepts of Biochemistry (for Physiotherapy and Pharmacy)
- Principles of Biochemistry (for Home Science and Nursing)

VIVA IN BIOCHEMISTRY

(Including Physiology, Molecular Biology & Biotechnology)

For the students of MBBS, MD, BDS, BMLT, DMLT, M.Sc. (Home Science), M.Sc. (Biochemistry), M.Sc. (Biotechnology), M.Sc. (Nursing), M.Sc. (Food Science & Technology), B.Sc. (Nursing), B.Sc. (Biochemistry), B.Sc. (Food Science & Technology) and other applied courses and

NEET & EXIT EXAMINATIONS

FIFTH EDITION

Prof. S.P. Singh
Ph.D., F.A.C.B.I.
Nominated by Govt. of India for **Medical Commonwealth Fellowship - 1983**
Cited in Wikipedia - **2010** for contribution to Biochemistry
Former **WHO Fellow** - Texas A & M University, Texas (U.S.A.) **- 1986**
Former **Prof. & Head Department of Biochemistry**
MLB Medical College, Jhansi - 284 128 (U.P.), India
and
Chief Consultant in Biochemistry
MLB Medical College and Associated Hospitals
Jhansi - 284 128 (U.P.), India

CBS
CBS Publishers & Distributors Pvt. Ltd.
New Delhi • Bengaluru • Chennai • Kochi • Kolkata • Mumbai
Hyderabad • Nagpur • Patna • Pune • Vijayawada

ISBN: 978-93-86478-61-0

First Edition: 1998
Second Edition: 2003
Third Edition: 2004
Fourth Edition: 2008
Fifth Edition: 2018
Reprint: 2020

Published by **Satish Kumar Jain** and produced by **Varun Jain** for
CBS Publishers & Distributors Pvt. Ltd.,
4819/XI Prahlad Street, 24 Ansari Road, Daryaganj, New Delhi - 110002
delhi@cbspd.com, cbspubs@airtelmail.in • www.cbspd.com
Ph.: 23289259, 23266861, 23266867 • Fax: 011-23243014

Corporate Office: 204 FIE, Industrial Area, Patparganj, Delhi - 110 092
Ph: 49344934 • Fax: 011-49344935
E-mail: publishing@cbspd.com • publicity@cbspd.com

Branches:

- ***Bengaluru:*** 2975, 17th Cross, K.R. Road, Bansankari 2nd Stage, Bengaluru - 70 • Ph: +91-80-26771678/79 • Fax: +91-80-26771680 E-mail: cbsbng@gmail.com, bangalore@cbspd.com
- ***Chennai:*** No. 7, Subbaraya Street, Shenoy Nagar, Chennai - 600030 Ph: +91-44-26681266, 26680620 • Fax: +91-44-42032115 E-mail: chennai@cbspd.com
- ***Kochi:*** Ashana House, 39/1904, A.M. Thomas Road, Valanjambalam, Ernakulum, Kochi • Ph: +91-484-4059061-65 Fax: +91-484-4059065 • E-mail: cochin@cbspd.com
- ***Kolkata:*** 6-B, Ground Floor, Rameshwar Shaw Road, Kolkata - 700014 Ph: +91-33-22891126/7/8 • E-mail: kolkata@cbspd.com
- ***Mumbai:*** 83-C, Dr. E. Moses Road, Worli, Mumbai - 400018 Ph: +91-9833017933, 022-24902340/41 • E-mail: mumbai@cbspd.com

Representatives:

- Hyderabad: 0-9885175004
- Patna: 0-9334159340
- Jharkhand: 0-9811541605
- Nagpur: 0-9021734563
- Pune: 0-9623451994
- Uttarakhand: 0-9716462459

Printed at: Neekunj Print Process, Delhi

Dedicated to

Shri Narendra Damodardas Ji Modi
Hon'ble & Very Dynamic Prime Minister of India

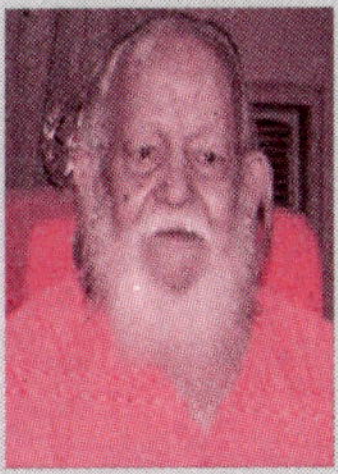

In the everlasting memory of, Late Shri Mahant Avaidyanathji, Gorakhnath Peeth, Gorakhpur, U.P (28/05/1921 to 12/09/2014), Ex- Parliamentarian.

Dr. R.K. Srivastava
M.S. (Ortho), D.N.B.
Ex. Director General Health Services, Govt. of India, New Delhi
&
Former President, Medical Council of India

Prof. Mridula Kapur
M.S., D.N.B., FAGS,
Ex-Professor & HOD Gynaecology Department
MLB Medical College, Jhansi

Prof. R.K. Gandhi
M.Sc., LL.B., M.D. (Forensic Medicine)
MLB Medical College, Jhansi

Prof. D.N. Mishra
M.D., D.N.B., F.C.C.P.
Medicine Department, MLB Medical College, Jhansi

Prof. Ajai Bhargava
Biochemistry Department, Jhalawar Medical College,
Jhalawar (Rajasthan)

Prof. Brijendra Singh
M.S. (Anatomy)
A.I.I.M.S., Jodhpur (Rajasthan)

Shri Raj Pratap Singh
Senior IAS, UP

Shri Sudhir Mahadeo Bobde
Senior IAS, UP

Preface to the Fifth Edition

It's a matter of great pleasure that **5th edition** of this book has come in the market at the demand of undergraduate and postgraduate students of Medical and Science faculties.

Students appearing for **NEET & EXIT Examinations** advised me to write such a book which may be useful for such entrances.

While writing this book, I have prepared it in such a way that it shall be of great worth upto their final MBBS examination and final M.D. examination of almost all the branches.

I accord my sincere thanks to my wife **Prof. Manju Singh,** Head, History Department, BKD Postgraduate College, Jhansi; my sons **Dr. Vikrant Singh**, **Er. Vijyant Singh**; **Smt. Charu Singh**, **Smt. Radha Singh** (Daughter-in-laws), **Ananya, Avvni** and **Kuhu** (my very very beloved grand Daughters), who all always encouraged me in finishing this book at the earliest possible.

Side-by-side, my sincere thanks to Dr. Jasbir Singh Parihar, Dr. Hari Madhav Sharan Yadav of Biochemistry Department, Sri. Vishan Lal (Ex. Librarian), MLB Medical College, Jhansi for their constant support in giving this book the present shape.

I am highly indebted to my well wishers, i.e., Sri Satish Kumar Jain, CMD, M/s. CBS Publishers & Distributors Pvt. Ltd., Mr. B.M. Singh, Mr. O N Nayar, Mr. J.K. Tiwari and Mr. Anurag Trivedi all associated with this group since long – who always support me for bringing new edition of books every year.

In the end, I am highly obliged to Mr. Prakash Sahu, for composing this book at an early date.

September, 2017 — S.P. Singh

PREFACE TO THE FIRST EDITION

Growing demand of the students led me to write the small book **'Viva in Biochemistry'** which in fact shall fulfill the desire of the students of medical, biotechnology, homoeopathic, agriculture and as well as general science students going through biochemistry.

While going to face viva-voce examination, it is never possible for the students to go through any text book because of its thickness. At this stage, they require a small cozy book in order to conceive the question with its answer within no time. Keeping this aspect in mind, the book has been written. Language of this book has been kept easily understandable.

I am really highly obliged to my wife Dr. (Smt.) Manju Singh, Reader, Bundelkhand College, Jhansi for her sincere encouragement in the write-up of this book. I am also highly indebted to my well wishers i.e., Prof. Mridula Kapur, Head, Department of Obstetrics & Gynaecology of MLB Medical College, Dr. K.P. Singh, Senior Surgeon, District Hospital, Jhansi, Prof R.K. Gandhi, Head, Department of Forensic Medicine, Dr. D.P. Singh Maurya, Department of Pharmacology, who all always pushed me to finish the gigantic work at the earliest possible.

I am also highly thankful for the sincere suggestions of my fellow colleagues i.e., Prof. S.D. Bhardwaj, Prof. V.D. Bohra, Prof. Praveen Sharma, Prof. Maheep Sinha (all of Jaipur) Prof. P.P. Singh (Udaipur), Prof. P.K. Sharma (Ajmer), Prof. C.R. Vyas (Bikaner), Prof. D.C. Sharma (Jaipur), Prof. Nisha Khalsa (Jodhpur), Prof. R.C. Gupta (Kota), Prof. R.K. Singh (Lucknow), Dr. V.K. Singh (Lucknow), Prof. V.S. Singh (Meerut), Dr. S.P. Saxena (Gorakhpur), Dr. Ajai Kumar (Kanpur), Prof R.K. Mittal (Allahabad), Dr. Geeta Jaiswal (Allahabad), Prof. M.C. Pant (Agra), Prof. A.K. Singh (Ranchi), Prof. B. Karr (Cuttack), Prof. L.M. Srivastava (New Delhi), Prof. A.G. Singh (Manipur), Prof. B.K.

Aggarwal (Bhopal), Prof. Meena Verma (Indore), Prof. B.L. Patel (Raipur), Prof. Sneh Shukla (Bhopal), Prof. Neelima Singh (Gwalior), Prof. Kiran Hasija (Jabalpur), Prof. N.K. Gandhi, Anaesthesia Department, S.N. Medical College, Agra, Dr. R.K. Srivastava, Medical Superintendent, Safdarjung Hospital, New Delhi, Prof. B.L. Verma, Dept. of P.S.M. (Jhansi), Dr. Kishan Lal Gupta (Jammu), Prof. Shamsuddin Bisati (Srinagar, J&K State), Dr. Vijai Anand, M.D. (Medicine), Meerut, Dr. Anil Kumar, Reader, Department of Genetic Engineering (Pantnagar University), Dr. Anshuman Singh (Pratapgarh), Dr. Krishna Dev Shakya, (Delhi) Mr. Bishan Lal, Librarian, Mr. Siddiqui Ali, Stenographer and the students community.

I am also highly grateful to my well wishers, i.e., Prof. P.L. Shukla, Retd. Principal and Dean, B.R.D. Medical College, Gorakhpur, UP, Journalists Shri Ramesh Chaube and Shri Arun Dwivedi of Jhansi, my brothers Shri C.P. Singh, Joint Director, Cement Research Institute of India, Ballabhgarh (Haryana), Shri. I.P. Singh, Works Manager, Northern Railway Workshop, Kalka (Haryana), Mr. V.P. Singh, Civil Defence Officer, Bareilly, Mr. Ajai Pal Singh and sister Shakuntala Devi (Bikaner), Mr Satish Kumar Jain and Mr. Vinod Kumar Jain of CBS Publishers & Distributors, New Delhi, who always thought very good of mine.

I shall fail in my duty if I do not express the sacrifice done by my sons i.e., Vikrant and Vijyant during write up of this book.

In the end suggestions from the readers and students shall be highly appreciated in order to improve this book further for the welfare of masses.

Dussehra 11th Oct' 97 **- S.P. Singh**
(The pious day on which
Lord Rama got victory over Ravana)

Contents

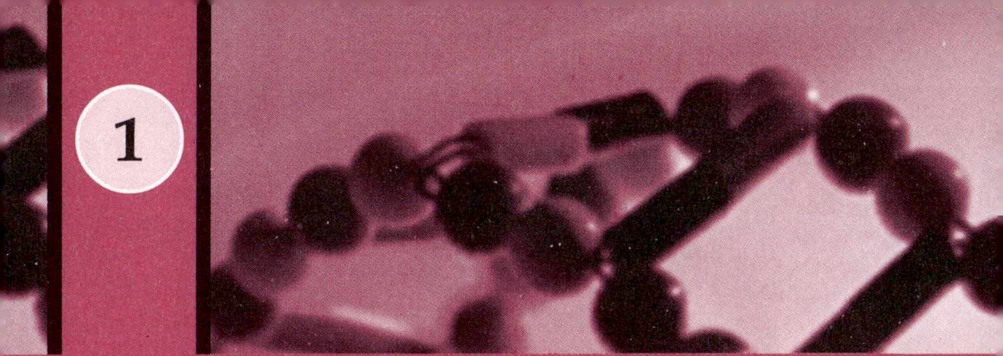

1

CARBOHYDRATES

Q.1. Define carbohydrates.

Ans. These may be defined as either polyhydric aldehydic or ketonic alcohols or their derivatives.

As the word **'carbohydrates'** indicates, these are the compounds usually made-up of carbon, hydrogen and oxygen, sometimes they may also contain nitrogen and sulphur in their molecules as in the case of higher carbohydrates like mucopolysaccharides (hyaluronic acid, chondroitin sulphates, heparin, etc.).

Q.2. Name the important carbohydrates.

Ans. Important examples include glucose, fructose, galactose, sucrose, starch and glycogen.

Q.3. Name the important hexoses.

Ans. Glucose, galactose, fructose and mannose.

Q.4. Name the important pentoses.

Ans. Ribose, ribulose, xylose and xylulose.

Q.5. Name the important tetroses.

Ans. Erythrose and erythrulose.

Q.6. Name the important trisaccharide.

Ans Raffinose.

Q.7. Which is the most important class of monosaccharides?

Ans. Hexoses.

Q.8. What is the classification of carbohydrates?

Ans. Carbohydrates have been classified into three main categories :

(a) Monosaccharides
(b) Oligosaccharides
(c) Polysaccharides

Q.9. What are oligosaccharides?

Ans. These are the carbohydrates made-up of 2-5 simple sugar units which include disaccharides, trisaccharides, and so on.

Q.10. What are polysaccharides?

Ans. These are the carbohydrates made-up of more than 5 simple sugar units which include starch, dextrins, glycogen, inulin etc.

Q.11. What are reducing sugars?

Ans. Reducing sugars are those which possess free aldehydic or ketonic group in their structures.

Q.12. What are epimers? Give examples.

Ans. Carbohydrates that differ in their configuration around a specific carbon atom other than the carboxyl carbon atom are called epimers. Glucose and galactose are epimers as they differ in their configuration around C-4 carbon atom. Similarly, glucose and mannose are epimers as they differ around C-2 carbon atom.

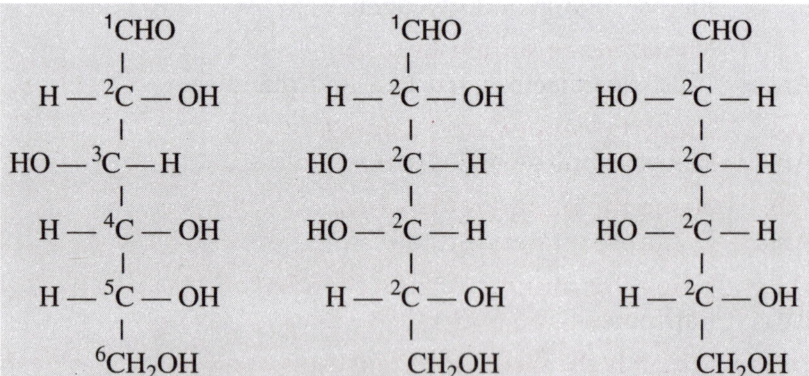

D - glucose D - galactose D - mannose

Q.13. How will you determine the D and L series of the sugars?

Ans. If the hydroxyl group on the highest asymmetric carbon atom is right oriented then the sugar belongs to D-series and if the hydroxyl group is left oriented then it belongs to L-series.

Q.14. What is mutarotation?

Ans. The change in specific rotation of an optically active solution without any change in other properties is known as mutarotation.

Q.15. Which property of reducing sugars best explains the ring or cyclic structure of the carbohydrates?

Ans. Mutarotation

Q.16. Which is the main sugar of the blood?

Ans. Glucose (dextrose)

Q.17. Is there any difference between glucose and dextrose?

Ans. No.

Q.18. What are anomers? Give examples.

Ans. Carbohydrates that differ only in their configuration around the carboxyl carbon atom are called anomers. The carboxyl carbon atom is called the anomeric carbon atom. α-D-glucose and β-D-glucose are the anomeric forms of D-glucose.

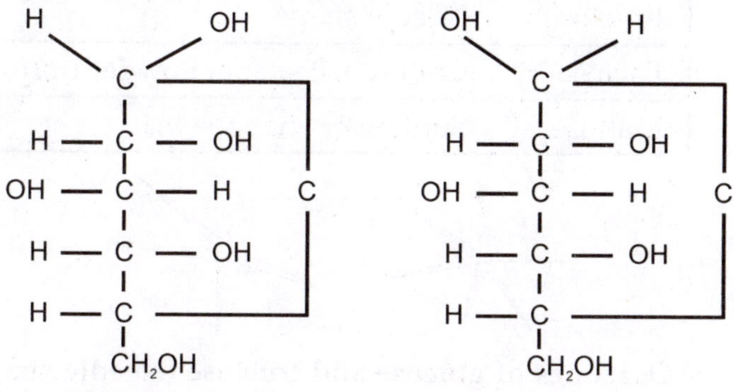

α-D-glucose β-D-glucose

Q.19. What is the percentage of glucose in honey?

Ans. 30-40%.

Q.20. What is another name of glucose?

Ans. Dextrose

Q.21. Which is the most important polysaccharide of the human body?

Ans. Glycogen.

Q.22. What are the components of lactose sugar?

Ans. Glucose and galactose.

Q.23. Draw the structure of L-glucose.

Ans.

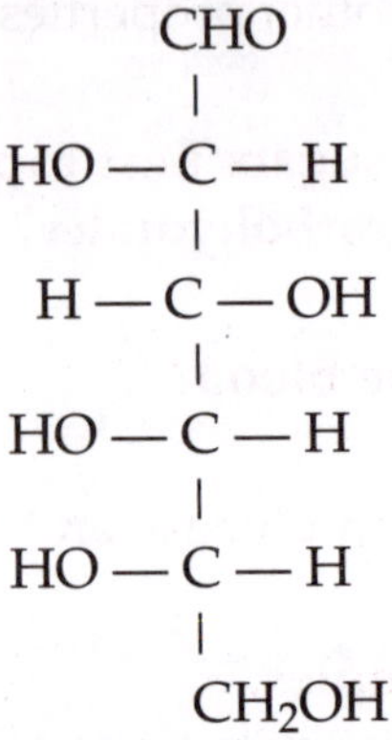

L-glucose

Q.24. What is the shape of osazones of glucose, fructose, lactose and maltose?

Ans.

Glucose :	Needle shape
Fructose :	Needle shape
Lactose :	Cotton ball shape/Powder puff shape
Maltose :	Sunflower shape

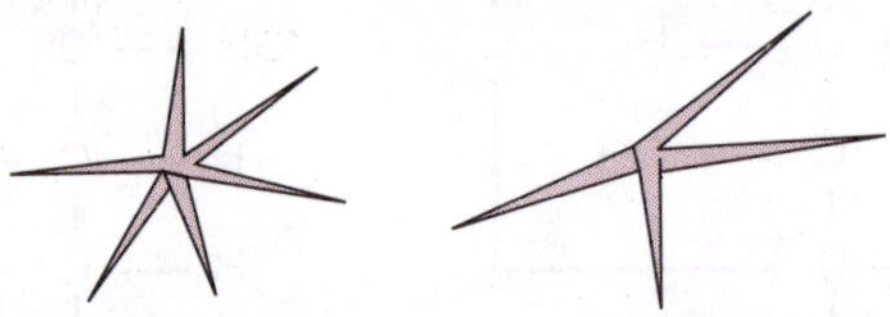

Osazones of glucose and fructose (Needle shaped)

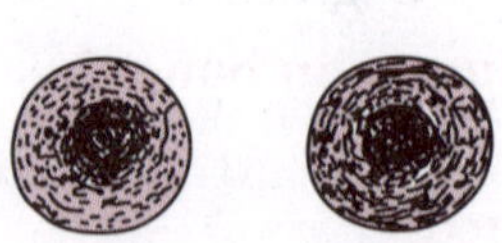

Osazones of lactose (Cotton ball or powder puff shaped)

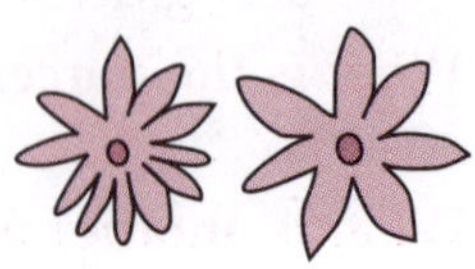

Osazones of maltose (Sunflower shaped)

Q.25. Why sucrose is a non-reducing sugar?

Ans. Sucrose sugar is made-up of one molecule each of glucose and fructose in which these remain linked to each other through the aldehyde group of glucose and keto group of fructose as a result of this linkage, both the reducing groups get blocked. Hence, sucrose is a non-reducing sugar.

Q.26. What is inversion?

Ans. The process by which dextrorotatory sucrose gets converted to a levorotatory mixture of glucose and fructose is called inversion.

$$\underset{(+65.5)}{\text{Sucrose}} \xrightarrow{H^+} \underset{(+52.7)}{\text{Glucose}} + \underset{(-92)}{\text{Fructose}}$$

Q.27. Why sucrose is called an invert sugar?

Ans. Sucrose upon hydrolysis yields glucose and fructose. Fructose has greater specific rotation than glucose. The resulting mixture is levorotatory. The mixture is known as invert sugar.

Q.28. What is the fate of sucrose when injected into the blood?

Ans. It will be excreted as such in the urine as there is no enzyme (sucrase) present in the blood to hydrolyze it.

Q.29. In which fluid lactose is found most?

Ans. Milk.

Q.30. What are the components of starch?

Ans. (a) Amylose (b) Amylopectin

Q.31. What is aglycone?

Ans. The non-carbohydrate portion of a glycoside is called aglycone.

Q.32. What are dextrins?

Ans. Dextrins are the partially degraded breakdown products of starch.

Q.33. What is the difference between starch and cellulose?

Ans. In starch, the glucose units remain linked by α (l, 4) glucosidic linkages, whereas in the cellulose, the glucose units remain linked by β (l, 4) glucosidic linkages.

Q.34. What is the difference between amylose and amylopectin?

Ans.

Amylose	Amylopectin
1. Low molecular weight (10,000-1,00,000)	1. High molecular weight (50,000-10,00,000)
2. About 3,00 glucose units	2. About 1,000 glucose units
3. 10-20% in starch	3. 80-90% in starch
4. Linear molecule containing α (1, 4) linkages	4. Branched molecules containing α (l, 4) and α (1, 6) linkages at branching site
5. Gives blue colour with iodine solution	5. Gives violet colour with iodine solution
6. Soluble in water	6. It's sparingly soluble in water

Q.35. Which polysaccharides are eaten mostly by the human beings? Name any two.

Ans. Starch and cellulose.

Q.36. Why cellulose is not utilized by the human body?

Ans. The enzyme responsible for the cleavage of β (l, 4) linkages in the cellulose molecule remains absent in the human beings. This enzyme is called cellulase, hence it is not utilized.

Q.37. What is the advantage of consuming cellulose in the diet by the human beings?

Ans. Cellulose contributes **'roughage'** to the fecal matter as a result of which there is comparatively less risk of gastrointestinal and colon cancers. Stool is also passed easily.

Q.38. Which is the most important carbohydrate for humans/ animals?

Ans. Glucose is the most important carbohydrate.

Q.39. Which is the most important monosaccharide?

Ans. Glucose (dextrose) is the most important monosaccharide.

Q.40. Which is the most important polysaccharide of human beings?

Ans. Glycogen.

Q.41. What is 'mannitol' which is transfused to the patients?

Ans. It is a sugar alcohol and is obtained by the reduction of mannose. It's structure is as follows:

CHO	CH_2OH
|	|
$(CHOH)_4$	$(CHOH)_4$
|	|
CH_2OH	CH_2OH
Mannose	Mannitol

Q.42. Give the structure of glucose and fructose.

Ans.

H—C=O	CH_2OH
|	|
H—C—OH	C=O
|	|
HO—C—H	HO—C—H
|	|
H—C—OH	H—C—OH
|	|
H—C—OH	H—C—OH
|	|
CH_2OH	CH_2OH
Glucose	Fructose

Q.43. What is the percentage of fructose in honey?

Ans. 30-40%

Q.44. Name some disaccharides.

Ans. Maltose, sucrose and lactose.

Q.45. Which disaccharides does mother's milk contain?

Ans. Lactose.

Q.46. How lactose is prepared commercially?

Ans. From milk.

Q.47. What is lactosuria?

Ans. Lactosuria is a pathological condition in which appreciable amount of lactose is found in the urine.

Q.48. Is there any difference between glycosuria and glucosuria?

Ans. No difference. They are synonymous words.

Q.49. What do you mean by glucosuria and glycosuria?

Ans. Both mean that the appreciable amount of glucose is appearing in the urine.

Q.50. What is fructosuria?

Ans. It's a pathological condition in which appreciable amount of fructose sugar appears in urine.

Q.51. What is galactosuria?

Ans. It's a pathological condition in which appreciable amount of galactose sugar appears in urine.

Q.52. What is saccharimeter?

Ans. It's an instrument with the help of which the extent of rotation of sugar solutions is determined.

Q.53. Name mucopolysaccharides.

Ans. Hyaluronic acid, chondroitin sulphates and heparin.

Q.54. What are the constituent units of sucrose?

Ans. Glucose and fructose.

Q.55. What is pentosuria?

Ans. It's a pathological state in which appreciable amount of pentose sugar appears in the urine.

It's also said to occur in normal individuals after the ingestion of large amount of certain fruits.

Q.56. Name any four homopolysaccharides?

Ans. Glycogen, starch, cellulose and inulin.

Q.57. Where is glycogen found in the human body?

Ans. Liver, muscles, kidney and other tissues but is not found in brain.

Q.58. Name any three heteropolysaccharides.

Ans. Hyaluronic acid, chondroitin sulphates and heparin.

Q.59. Name any carbohydrate which acts as an anticoagulant.

Ans. Heparin.

Q.60. Can you name any such polysaccharide which may be used as a plasma substitute?

Ans. Dextran.

Q.61. What are the substances that give false Benedict's test?

Ans. Large concentration of uric acid, creatinine, salicylates (aspirin), vitamin C, etc.

Q.62. What is the difference between Benedict's Qualitative test and Barfoed's test?

Ans. ***Benedict's qualitative test*** is a reduction test carried out in the alkaline medium whereas **Barfoed's test** is a reduction test carried out in acidic medium.

Q.63. What is the general test for carbohydrates?

Ans. Molisch test.

Q.64. What is the first breakdown product of glycogen metabolism?

Ans. Glucose-1-phosphate.

Q.65. Name the vitamin whose structure closely resembles that of a monosaccharide?

Ans. Vitamin C (ascorbic acid)

Q.66. From nutrition point of view, which carbohydrate is of importance for infants?

Ans. Lactose (found in milk)

Q.67. What is the importance of hyaluronic acid?

Ans. It is the ground substance of synovial fluid of joints and serves as lubricant and shock absorbent in joints which otherwise become dry and create a sound which one can hear easily.

Q.68. Name any two amino sugars.

Ans. Glucosamine and galactosamine.

Q.69. Name complex carbohydrate derivatives.

Ans. Sialic acid and muramic acid.

Q.70. Define glycoconjugates

Ans. These may be referred to as the carbohydrates which are found in combination with a non-carbohydrate moiety.

Q.71. What is the main property of pectins?

Ans. They are used as **gelling agent,** particularly in Jams, Jellies and Marmalades.

Q.72. Which sugar is the energy source of sperms?

Ans. Fructose.

Q.73. Who discovered and in which year that fructose is the source of energy for sperms?

Ans. Scientist Thaddeus Mann in the year 1975.

Q.74. What is the temperature required for normal sperm production?

Ans. It's about 2-3°C below core body temperature.

Q.75. What's the sperm range when one is called as infertile?

Ans. Less than 20 millions/ml.

Q.76. What is the pH of semen?

Ans. 7.2 - 7.7

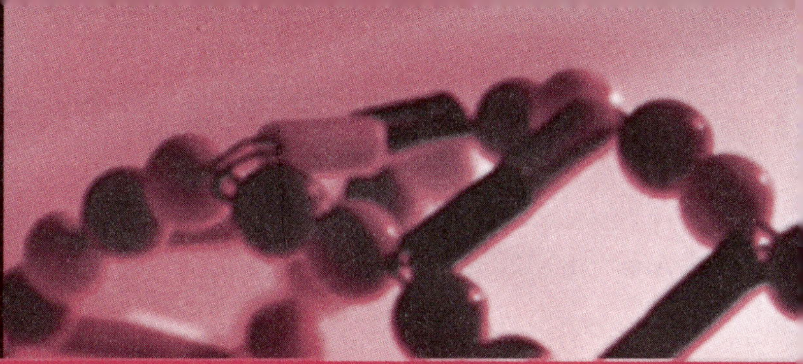

2

Carbohydrates Metabolism

Q.1. What are the various pathways by which glucose is utilised?

Ans.
1. Glycolysis followed by Tricarboxylic acid cycle
2. Hexose monophosphate shunt pathway
3. Glycogenesis (synthesis of glycogen from glucose)
4. Conversion to galactose and then to lactose
5. Conversion to fat
6. Gives rise to non-essential amino acids

Q.2. Which is the main sugar of the blood?

Ans. Glucose

Q.3. Is glucose easily permeable through the cellular membrane?

Ans. Yes

Q.4. Is liver or muscle glycogen easily available for metabolism?

Ans. Liver glycogen

Q.5. What is glycolysis?

Ans. Breakdown of glucose or glycogen to pyruvic acid or lactic acid is called glycolysis.

Q.6. What is the key enzyme of glycolytic pathway?

Ans. Phosphofructokinase (PFK).

Q.7. What is the range of fasting blood sugar?

Ans. 70-100 mg/dl. (4.2 - 6.1 mmol/l)

Q.8. What is the normal blood sugar level?

Ans. 80-120 mg/dl.

Q.9. What is the range of postprandial (PP) blood sugar level?

Ans. Less than 140 mg/dl.

Q.10. What is the normal range of renal threshold value for glucose?

Ans. 160-180 mg/dl.

Q.11. What is the ATP yield per molecule of glucose oxidised in glycolysis *under anaerobic conditions?*

Ans. Two ATP per molecule of glucose metabolized.

Q.12. What is the ATP yield per molecule of glycosyl unit of glycogen oxidised in glycolysis under *anaerobic conditions?*

Ans. Three

Q.13. What is the ATP yield per molecule (one molecule) of glucose if oxidised completely via glycolysis and TCA cycle under aerobic conditions?

Ans. 32 ATP per molecule of glucose oxidised i.e., via glycolysis 12 ATP and via TCA cycle 20 ATP.

Q.14. How many molecules of ATP are formed in TCA cycle from (i) one molecule of acetyl CoA, and (ii) one molecule of pyruvate?

Ans. (i) 10 ATP (ii) 12.5 ATP

Q.15. What is the generation of ATP through pyruvate dehydrogenase reaction alone by 2 moles of pyruvic acid?

Ans. 5

Q.16. What is the generation of ATP in TCA cycle alone?

Ans. 10+10 = 20 ATP.

Q.17. How many molecules of ATP are generated upon oxidation of one molecule of NADH via electron transport chain (ETC)?

Ans. 2.5

Q.18. How many molecules of ATP are generated upon oxidation of one molecule of FADH via electron transport chain (ETC)?

Ans. 1.5

Q.19. What is the full form of TCA cycle?

Ans. Tri-carboxylic acid cycle.

Q.20. What is another name of TCA cycle?

Ans. Citric acid cycle.

Q.21. What is yet another name of TCA cycle?

Ans. Krebs cycle.

Q.22. Who invented TCA cycle?

Ans. Sir Hans Krebs (Nobel Prize in 1953)

Q.23. What is the chemical structure of Tricarboxylic acid?

Ans.

$$\begin{array}{c} CH_2 - COOH \\ | \\ HO - C - COOH \\ | \\ CH_2 - COOH \end{array}$$

Q.24. What do you know about the amphibolic nature (biological significance) of TCA cycle?

Ans. TCA cycle is both **catabolic** and **anabolic** in nature, therefore, regarded **as amphibolic.** For example, most amino acids enter the cycle via intermediates and get oxidized (catabolism). Side-by-side, the intermediates of TCA cycle are useful for biosynthetic reactions (anabolism), e.g. succinyl CoA in the synthesis of heme; oxaloacetate and α-ketoglutarate for the formation of aspartate and glutamate respectively.

Q.25. Where does substrate level phosphorylation occur in TCA cycle?

Ans. In the conversion of succinyl CoA to succinate, the reaction is catalysed by the enzyme succinate thiokinase, GTP is formed which, in turn, gets converted to ATP.

Q.26. Name any dicarboxylic acid.

Ans. Succinic acid.

Q.27. What is the chemical structure of succinic acid?

Ans.

$$\begin{array}{l} CH_2COOH \\ | \\ CH_2COOH \end{array}$$

Q.28. Name two keto acids involved in carbohydrate metabolism?

Ans. (i) Pyruvic acid

(ii) α-ketoglutaric acid.

Q.29. What is oxidative decarboxylation?

Ans. Oxidation accompanied by decarboxylation is called oxidative decarboxylation.

Q.30. Why TCA cycle is considered to be the common pathway for carbohydrate, lipid and protein metabolism?

Ans. It's considered to be the common pathway for the metabolism of carbohydrates, lipids and proteins because it brings about complete oxidation of acetyl CoA to carbon dioxide and water.

Acetyl CoA is produced from all the three main metabolism:

Carbohydrate metabolism	: via	glycolysis
Lipid metabolism	: via	β-oxidation
Protein metabolism	: via	transamination

Q.31. What is the oxidative decarboxylation product of pyruvic acid?

Ans. Acetyl CoA

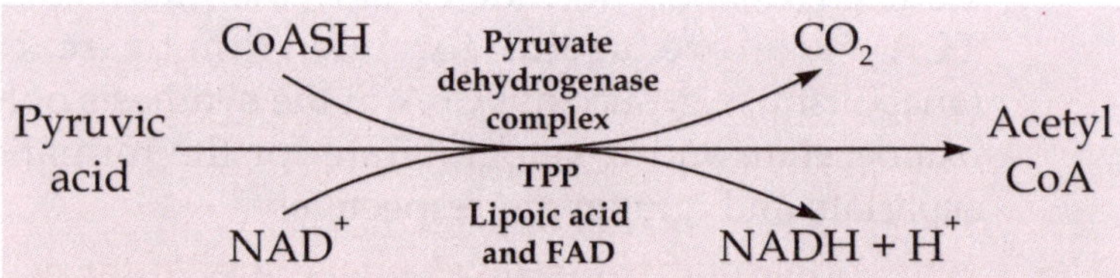

Q.32. Name the enzyme of the above oxidative decarboxylation reaction.

Ans. Pyruvate dehydrogenase complex. This is an enzyme complex which consists of the following three enzymes :

(i) Pyruvate dehydrogenase

(ii) Dihydro lipoyl transacetylase

(iii) Dihydro lipoyl dehydrogenase

Q.33. Which enzyme catalyzes the conversion of acetyl CoA to citric acid?

Ans. Citrate synthetase (condensing enzyme).

Q.34. Name the coenzymes and cofactors involved in the oxidative decarboxylation of pyruvic acid.

Ans.
1. Thiamine pyrophosphate (TPP)
2. Lipoic acid
3. Flavin adenine dinucleotide (FAD)
4. Nicotinamide adenine dinucleotide (NAD^+)
5. Coenzyme A (CoA-SH)
6. Mg^{++} ions

Q.35. Name the vitamin involved in the oxidative decarboxylation of pyruvic acid.

Ans. Lipoic acid.

Q.36. What is the other name of lipoic acid?

Ans. Thioctic acid.

Q.37. Which is the main site of carbohydrate metabolism?

Ans. Liver.

Q.38. Where does TCA cycle occur in the cell?

Ans. Mitochondria.

Q.39. Why it is called citric acid cycle or TCA cycle or Krebs cycle?

Ans. Because citric acid is formed first of all in this pathway. TCA- because the citric acid consists of three carboxylic groups.

Q.40. What is the importance/metabolic significance of hexose monophosphate shunt (HMP shunt) pathway?

Ans.
1. Provides NADPH which is used for the biosynthesis of fatty acids, steroids and other important substances of the body.
2. Provides pentose sugars which are used in the biosynthesis of nucleic acids.

Q.41. Name the sites of HMP shunt pathway.

Ans. Liver, adipose tissue, lactating mammary glands, adrenal cortex, testis, etc.

Q.42. What do you understand by branching and debranching enzymes?

Ans. Branching enzymes produce a branching in the molecule by establishing (l, 6) glycosidic linkages.

Debranching enzymes produce cleavage of α (1, 6) linkages.

Q.43. Name two reactions catalysed by kinases.

Ans. (i) $\text{Glucose} \xrightarrow{\text{Glucokinase}} \text{Glucose-6-PO}_4$

(ii) $\text{Fructose-6-PO}_4 \xrightarrow{\text{PFK}} \text{Fructose 1, 6-diPO}_4$

Q.44. Name two reactions catalysed by mutases.

Ans. (i) $\text{3-Phosphoglycerate} \xrightarrow[\text{mutase}]{\text{Phosphoglycerate}} \text{2-Phosphoglycerate}$

(ii) $\text{Glucose-1-PO}_4 \xrightarrow{\text{Phosphoglucomutase}} \text{Glucose-6-PO}_4$

Q.45. What is glycogenolysis?

Ans. It is the breakdown of polysaccharide glycogen into glucose in liver and kidney tissues and glucose-6-PO_4 in the muscles.

Q.46. Why is glucose-6-PO_4 end product of glycogenolysis in muscles?

Ans. Because muscles lack the enzyme glucose-6-phosphatase.

$$\text{Glucose-6-PO}_4 \xrightarrow{\text{Glucose-6-phosphatase}} \text{Glucose}$$

Q.47. Name the sites of glycogenolysis.

Ans. Main sites are liver and muscles.

Q.48. What is the role of cyclic AMP in glycogenolysis?

Ans. Cyclic AMP in the presence of dephosphophosphorylase kinase brings about the conversion of dephosphophosphorylase (inactive form) into phosphophosphorylase (active form).

Q.49. From where cyclic AMP comes in 'glycogenolysis'?

Ans. From ATP.

$$\text{ATP} \xrightarrow[\text{Mg}^{++}]{\text{adenyl cyclase}} \text{Cyclic AMP}$$

Q.50. What are the breakdown products of glycogen?

Ans. $\text{Glycogen} \xrightarrow{\text{Phosphorylase, Pi}} \text{Glucose-1-PO}_4$

$$\text{Glucose-1-PO}_4 \xrightarrow[\text{G-1, 6 diphosphate}]{\text{Phosphoglucomutase}} \text{Glucose-6-PO}_4$$

$$\text{Glucose-6-PO}_4 \xrightarrow{\text{Glucose-6-phosphatase}} \text{Glucose + Pi}$$

Q.51. What is the first breakdown product of glycogen metabolism?

Ans. Glucose-1-phosphate

Q.52. What is gluconeogenesis? Name some gluconeogenic substances.

Ans. It is the formation of glucose or glycogen from non-carbohydrate sources like glycerol, lactic acid, propionic acid, pyruvic acid and amino acids.

Q.53. What is the difference between gluconeogenesis and neoglucogenesis?

Ans. No difference

Q.54. Name the main sites of gluconeogenesis.

Ans. Liver and kidneys.

Q.55. Name some gluconeogenic amino acids.

Ans. Glycine, valine, methionine, cysteine, aspartic acid and glutamic acid.

Q.56. What is the significance of 'gluconeogenesis pathway?

Ans. (i) It's a useful pathway especially when an individual is consuming less carbohydrates.

(ii) It helps in the maintenance of blood sugar level within its normal range.

(iii) It brings about proper disposal of glycerol and lactic acid, which are formed during muscular activity/ exercise.

Q.57. Are there other alternative pathways of carbohydrate metabolism than the glycolysis and TCA cycle?

Ans. Following are the other two alternative pathways of carbohydrate metabolism.

(i) Pentose phosphate pathway (HMP shunt or phosphogluconate oxidative pathway or Warburg-Dickens-Lipmann pathway).

(ii) Glucuronic acid cycle.

Q.58. What happens if carbohydrates are taken in excess?

Ans. Excess intake of carbohydrates is harmful because in the animal body excess carbohydrates are converted to fats which are eventually stored in various tissues of the body causing development of obesity.

Q.59. Are there found other monosaccharides than glucose in the blood?

Ans. Ordinarily other monosaccharides like galactose, fructose and mannose do not remain present in the blood because all these have a tendency to be converted to glucose by their metabolisms respectively. They may be found to be present in the blood only if their metabolism gets defected.

Q.60. Are there present oligosaccharides or polysaccharides in the blood?

Ans. No, because all oligosaccharides and polysaccharides after digestion and metabolism are converted into glucose.

Q.61. How blood sugar level is controlled within its normal limits?

Ans. It is kept controlled within its normal range by the liver mainly by balance between glycogenesis and glycogenolysis-cum-gluconeogenesis. Besides these, several other factors like hormones, kidneys etc. do also play role.

Q.62. Name the enzymes responsible for the reversal of glycolysis i.e. gluconeogenesis pathway.

Ans. (i) Pyruvate carboxylase

(ii) Phosphoenolpyruvate carboxykinase

(iii) Fructose 1, 6-diphosphatase

(iv) Glucose-6-phosphatase

Q.63. What is Cori's cycle?

Ans. Lactic acid produced in the muscles reaches the liver through blood where it's converted to glucose by gluconeogenesis which again becomes a source of energy for utilization. This process continues in a cyclic manner as shown below and is called **'Cori's cycle'.**

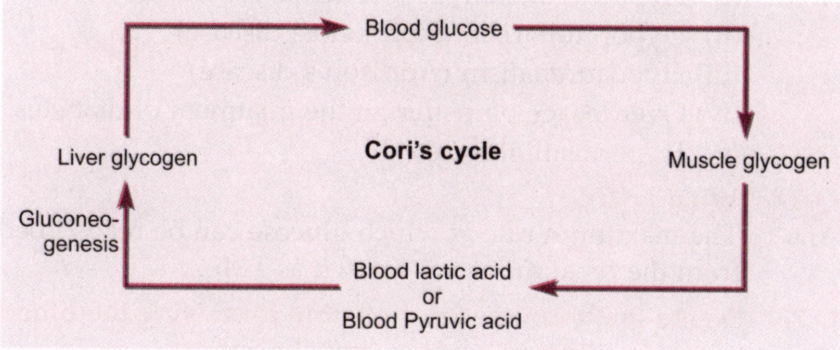

Q.64. How pyruvate is converted to glucose?

Ans. Pyruvate gets converted to glucose by the pathway of gluconeogenesis as shown below :

Pyruvate ⟶ Oxaloacetate

Oxaloacetate ⟶ Phosphoenolpyruvate

Phosphoenolpyruvate ⟶ Glucose

Q.65. What is true glucose?

Ans. True glucose means glucose alone without taking into account the presence of any other reducing substances in the blood.

Q.66. How will you estimate true glucose (tell the best method)?

Ans. (i) GOD/POD method (glucose oxidase peroxidase method).

(ii) Nelson-Somogyi method (it's as accurate as enzymic method but time consuming).

(iii) O-toluidine method.

Q.67. Name the conditions/diseases in which blood sugar level gets increased (elevated).

Ans. (i) Diabetes mellitus

(ii) Hyperpituitarism

(iii) Hyperthyroidism

(iv) Hyperadrenalism

(v) Thyrotoxicosis

Q.68. Name the conditions/diseases in which blood sugar level is found to be low.

Ans. (i) Hypothyroidism (myxoedema, cretinism)
(ii) Hypopituitarism (Simmonds' disease)
(iii) Hypoadrenalism (Addison's disease)
(iv) Overdosage of insulin in the treatment of diabetes.
(v) Hyperinsulinism, etc.

Q.69. What is TM_G?

Ans. The maximum rate at which glucose can be reabsorbed from the renal tubules is known as TM_G.

Q.70. Name the hormones responsible for raising the blood sugar level i.e. hyperglycaemic hormones.

Ans. (i) Glucagon
(ii) Epinephrine
(iii) Thyroid hormones
(iv) Adrenal cortex hormones
(v) Growth hormone etc.

Q.71. What is diabetes mellitus?

Ans. A state of constant hyperglycaemia is known as diabetes mellitus which takes place due to the deficiency of insulin hormone.

Q.72. What is the literal meaning of dia, betes and mellitus?

Ans. Diabetes comes from Greek word which means:
Dia = through, betes = passing, mellitus = honey (sweet)
मधुमेह (मधु + मेह या मधु + बारिश अर्थात मूत्र के द्वारा शहद अर्थात शक्कर की बारिश); ऐसे रोगी जिन्हें मधुमेह होती है, वे यदि पक्के फर्श पर मूत्र त्याग करते हैं तो थोड़ी ही देर में उस स्थान पर चीटे आ जाते हैं जो कि इस प्रकार से मूत्र के माध्यम से त्यागी गई शक्कर को ग्रहण करते हैं। यह शक्कर उन्हें ऊर्जा प्रदान करती है।

Q.73. What is hypoglycaemia?

Ans. A state in which blood sugar level gets lowered than the normal range.

Q.74. What is hyperglycaemia?

Ans. A state in which blood sugar level gets raised than the normal range.

Q.75. What is insulin?

Ans. It's a hypoglycaemic hormone.

Q.76. Who discovered the existence of insulin?

Ans. Banting, Best and Macleod in the year 1921.

Q.77. Who discovered the structure of insulin?

Ans. **Sanger,** for which he was awarded **Nobel Prize** in the year **1958**. (Sanger won the **Nobel Prize** twice i.e., in **1958** for discovering the **structure of protein Insulin** and in **1980** for the **base sequence of nucleic acids**).

Q.78. From where insulin is secreted in the human body?

Ans. By the β-cells of the islets of Langerhans of the pancreas.

Q.79. What do you know about the structure of insulin hormone?

Ans. It is a polypeptide and consists of 51 amino acids. It consists of two chains i.e. 'A' and 'B'. 'A' chain contains 21 whereas 'B' 30 amino acids. Both these chains remain linked to each other by two interchain disulfide bridges that connect A7 to B7 and A20 to B19. A third interchain disulfide bridge connects residues 6 and 11 of the A chain.

Q.80. Why insulin cannot be given orally to the diabetic patients?

Ans. Insulin (proteinous in nature) is a polypeptide which may be easily digested by the proteolytic enzymes of the digestive system into amino acids before it reaches the blood, hence it's not given orally (by mouth).

Q.81. What is diabetes insipidus?

Ans. Lack of anti-diuretic hormone (ADH) gives rise to a condition known as diabetes insipidus. Level of sugar in blood of such individuals is found within normal range **but such individuals may excrete urine upto 30 litres per day.**

Q.82. What is the abnormality in the urine samples of severe diabetic patient versus starving individual?

Ans. In severe diabetic patient, urine will exhibit the presence of sugar and ketone bodies whereas in case of starving individuals only ketone bodies will be found and no sugar.

Q.83. Which different reducing sugars appear in urine and under what conditions?

Ans.

Glucose : **(glucosuria)**.	Appears in urine in **renal glycosuria** and diabetes mellitus.
Lactose : **(lactosuria)**	During later stage of pregnancy and lactation.
Galactose: **(galactosuria)**	In galactosaemia due to the deficiency of enzyme galactose–1–PO_4 uridyl transferase. This condition is found in infants.
Fructose : **(fructosuria)**	Due to consumption of large amount of fruits containing fructose such as plums, cherry, grapes, etc.
Pentoses : **(pentosuria)**	Due to consumption of large amount of fruits containing pentoses. Also, in congenital abnormality characterized by inability to metabolize L-xylulose.

Q.84. How the collection of blood specimen is done for estimating blood glucose?

Ans. Blood sample is collected in potassium oxalate-sodium fluoride vial, popularly known as **'fluoride vial'.**

Q.85. What's the function of potassium oxalate and NaF in the vial?

Ans. (i) Potassium oxalate : Acts as an anticoagulant.

(ii) NaF : Prevents glycolysis by inhibiting the enzyme **enolase** of the **glycolytic pathway.**

Q.86. What is diabetic acidosis?

Ans. It is a state in which one finds elevated level of ketone bodies in the blood (ketonaemia) along with uncontrolled diabetes mellitus.

Q.87. What is the treatment of Favism?

Ans. Diet devoid of fava-beans.

Q.88. What is the treatment of diabetes mellitus?

Ans. (i) Oral administration of antidiabetic drugs.

(ii) Subcutaneous injection of soluble insulin.

(iii) Carbohydrates restricted diet and intake of fenugreek (methi) seeds powder (1–4 tea spoons per day depending upon the severity) is also helpful in controlling it.

(iv) Physical exercises like morning walk, and '**yoga**' are also helpful **(life-style changes)**.

Q.89. What is the role of isotonic $CuSO_4$ solution while estimating sugar in the blood?

Ans. It prevents the hemolysis of RBCs so that the glutathione which remains present in RBCs does not come out, which otherwise will also reduce the alkaline $CuSO_4$ and give rise to high blood sugar values.

Q.90. Of which pathway glucose-6-phosphate dehydrogenase is an important enzyme?

Ans. Pentose phosphate pathway

Q.91. What harm does the genetic deficiency of glucose-6-phosphate dehydrogenase cause?

Ans. Hemolysis and jaundice, particularly after the administration of vitamin K, sulpha drugs and quinine and after eating fava-beans.

Q.92. Which Indian races are susceptible to the genetic deficiency of glucose-6-phosphate dehydrogenase?

Ans. Parsis of Western India, Punjabis and Sindhis (P, P, S).

Q.93. What is Favism?

Ans. It's caused after eating Fava-beans (contains toxic substances) in which there occurs hemolysis as in such patients there is found genetic deficiency of enzyme glucose-6-phosphate dehydrogenase.

Q.94. What does the symbol ~P~ denote?

Ans. High energy phosphate group or bond.

Q.95. Who introduced the above symbol?

Ans. Scientist **Lipmann.**

Q.96. What's renal diabetes?

Ans. This is not the true diabetes. It's a very rare condition in which renal absorption of glucose gets so diminished that significant amount of glucose escapes into the urine. Such a condition is known as **renal diabetes.**

Q.97. How 'carbohydrate metabolism' is controlled in the human body?

Ans. It's controlled by a battery of hormones which are secreted from several endocrine glands for e.g., the pancreas, the anterior pituitary gland, and the adrenal cortex.

Q.98. What is insulin shock?

Ans. Administration of insulin to a normal animal leads to a profound hypoglycaemia resulting into convulsions or unconsciousness, such a state is termed as insulin shock.

Q.99. What do you mean by 'Antibodies' to insulin?

Ans. The repeated injection of insulin results in the production of antibodies to insulin in all the subjects, whether diabetic or not, after two or three months of treatment. At times, high concentrations of the antibodies may be found in such subjects, who are said to be ***'resistant to insulin'*** as insulin has got almost negligible effect in them.

Q.100. What is the effect of carbohydrate free diet in human beings?

Ans. Normally, ketone bodies are the normal end products of the fatty acids oxidation in the liver but the amount formed is relatively too small to be detected in the urine. But when the diet is carbohydrate free, ketosis takes place which is due to the fact that in the absence of carbohydrates, more fats (reserved in various tissues) burn (i.e. get oxidized) giving rise to more ketone bodies which are easily detectable in the urine (ketonuria).

Q.101. What is the other name of acetoacetic acid?

Ans. Diacetic acid.

Q.102. What is the normal level of ketone bodies in the blood?

Ans. Upto 3 mg per 100 ml.

Q.103. What is the level of ketone bodies in the blood of uncontrolled diabetes?

Ans. It may reach 300-400 mg/dl or even higher.

Q.104. What is the normal level of ketone bodies (as acetone) in the urine per day?

Ans. Upto 50 mg daily.

Q.105. What is the level of ketone bodies (as acetone) in the urine of uncontrolled diabetics per day?

Ans. 10-50g per litre may be found.

Q.106. What is diabetes insipidus?

Ans. The posterior pituitary secretes an antidiuretic hormone (ADH) named as pitressin, which is responsible to regulate the absorption of water by the renal tubules. Deficiency of this hormone leads to the condition known as **"diabetes insipidus"** in which enormous volume of urine is excreted **(upto 30 litres per 24 hrs.)** having a **sp.gr. of 1.001 to 1.003.**

Q.107. What is juvenile onset type diabetes?

Ans. The condition usually develops during the childhood and adulthood i.e. below 40 years of age in the subjects of normal body weight or less than that. Majority develops severe symptoms of diabetes mellitus acutely over a period of several weeks or months and if treatment with insulin is delayed, they may develop **ketoacidosis and diabetic coma.** Insulin administration in such cases is essential for their survival as the secretion of insulin is very poor in such cases. β-cells soon become exhausted of insulin and the cells become atrophied resulting in total diabetes mellitus.

Q.108. What is adult or maturity-onset type diabetes mellitus?

Ans. It usually develops in middle-aged or elderly subjects over the age of 40 years who are often obese. This is a mild or moderate type of diabetes which can be **controlled by diet and oral hypoglycaemic drugs.** In such cases, plasma insulin levels are low than the normal.

Q.109. Which compound do the patients of carcinoid, a tumour of the argentaffin cells of the pancreas secrete in large amount?

Ans. Serotonin

Q.110. If you get blue colour in the test tube while performing Benedict's qualitative test in an urine sample, then, how much concentration of sugar does it denote?

Ans. Almost nil i.e; negative test-which means of no significance.

Q.111. If you get greenish colour in the above test, then, how much concentration of sugar does it denote?

Ans. 0.5%

Q.112. If you get yellowish colour in the above test, then, how much concentration of sugar does it denote?

Ans. 1%

Q.113. If you get orangish colour in the above test, then, how much concentration of sugar does it denote?

Ans. 1.5%

Q.114. If you get reddish colour in the above test, then, how much concentration of sugar does it denote?

Ans. 2% and above.

Q.115. By using which drug experimental glycosuria may be induced in animals?

Ans. Phlorhizin or alloxan or streptozotocin.

Q.116. By using which drug experimental diabetes mellitus may be induced in animals?

Ans. Alloxan

Q.117. How much glucose may be excreted in the urine of a normal person in 24 hours?

Ans. Usually less than 100 mg

Q.118. How much glucose may be excreted in the urine of a severe diabetic person in 24 hours?

Ans. 5-6% or even more.

Q.119. Which enzyme is supposed to play role in the reabsorption of sugar in the renal tubules?

Ans. Phosphorylase.

Q.120. Name the conditions of endocrine hyperactivity in which one can find glucose in ones urine.

Ans. (a) hyperthyroidism
(b) hyperpituitarism
(c) hyperadrenalism

Q.121. What is the best mean (technique) of showing the presence of the minimum quantity of galactose in the urine of an individual?

Ans. Thin layer chromatography (TLC)

Q.122. Does anaesthesia cause raise in blood sugar level?

Ans. Yes

Q.123. Name the eatables which are supposed to be rich in fructose.

Ans. Fruits, honey, syrup and jams.

Q.124. Which enzyme is found to be lacking/absent in essential fructosuria?

Ans. Fructokinase

Q.125. What is the function of enzyme fructokinase?

Ans. It catalyses the conversion of fructose to fructose–1-phosphate

Q.126. Which enzyme is found to be lacking/missing in hereditary fructose intolerance?

Ans. Fructose–1–phosphate aldolase.

Q.127. What are the renal threshold values for galactose, fructose and pentoses?

Ans. They have no renal threshold, therefore, they are excreted in the urine as soon as there is an appreciable amount present in the blood.

Q.128. How many people in India are sufferers of diabetes mellitus today?

Ans. It is estimated that 5-6 crores Indians do have diabetes and the incidence is on increase.

Q.129. What are the main outside contributing factors of diabetes mellitus?

Ans.
- (i) Changed life style
- (ii) Eating habits
- (iii) Added stress, and
- (iv) Reduced physical exercises

Q.130. What are the major types of diabetes?

Ans.
- (a) Type I diabetes (earlier also known as Insulin Dependent Diabetes)
- (b) Type II diabetes (Insulin Independent Diabetes)
- (c) Gestational diabetes (**diabetes which is caused during pregnancy**)

Q.131. How is diabetes diagnosed?

Ans. Blood sugar test is performed in clinical laboratories on patients who are suspected to have diabetes. The tests are known as :

FBS – Fasting Blood Sugar

PPBS – Post-Prandial Blood Sugar

(Post-prandial means 2 hrs after lunch or meal or 75 g. glucose load)

RBS – Random Blood Sugar

Elevated blood sugar levels (far higher than the normal) suggest that the patient has an impaired glucose metabolism. Then the doctor correlates certain clinical symptoms and concludes that it is diabetes.

Q.132. What is the cause of diabetes mellitus?

Ans. Insulin is a hormone secreted by the pancreas, which is vital in glucose metabolism. Insulin attaches itself to the cell surface (insulin receptors) and pumps the glucose molecule inside the cell for the cell's metabolic need. Therefore, any hinderance in insulin production (from pancreas) in its quantity or quality may result in failure of promoting glucose metabolism. In good number of diabetic patients, it has been observed that glucose metabolism is impaired even in the presence of enough quantity of insulin, thereby suggesting that the insulin receptors have become insensitive. The inability due to either of the problems results in hyperglycaemia (hyper = excess; glycaemia = sugar level).

Q.133. How is diabetes controlled?

Ans. The objective of treatment for diabetes is to bring down the blood glucose level as close as possible to the normal range. This is achieved by the following three major ways:

(a) Following a strict diet protocol

(b) Adhering to routine and uniform physical exercises

(c) Taking medicines and/or injections to control the blood sugar levels

Q.134. What is glycated or glycosylated (HbA_1c) haemoglobin test?

Ans. HbA_1c test is a laboratory procedure which estimates the portion of haemoglobin that has been glycated. The word glycated means that the sugar has been added. **In a normal individual 5-6% of the haemoglobin molecule should be glycated. However, in uncontrolled diabetic patient the levels can go even more than 20% which indicates that the patients has an uncontrolled hyperglycaemia.** Because daily blood glucose testing provides only a snapshot of glycaemic control at the moment of test, it varies a lot day-to-day, and at times moment-to-moment. Thus, the patient and the doctor are unsure about the glycaemic control when only blood glucose levels are relied upon. On the other hand, as haemoglobin has a life span of 120 days, HbA_1c test reveals the **glycaemic control** over a period of last 3 months without getting "influenced" like that of blood sugar. To make it little clear to understand, blood sugar levels are like individual scores of cricket batsman, whereas, HbA_1c test results are like his batting average.

Q.135. What is the importance of HbA_1c in glycaemic control?

Ans. (a) To confirm consistencies or highlight discrepancies between blood glucose self-monitoring results produced by the patients and the actual degree of overall control.

(b) In differentiating stress induced, transient glucose irregularities from true diabetes.

(c) Most useful in evaluating the initial 1-2 months of diabetic control in a newly pregnant diabetic female, significant elevation is often predictive of congenital anomalies.

(d) As a risk factor for the development of tissue complications as per the results of DCCT (Diabetes control and complications trial).

Q.136. What are the complications (metabolic abnormalities) of uncontrolled diabetes mellitus?

Ans. The HbA_1c test results correlate well with that of the real glycaemic control and significant reductions in HbA_1c levels result in reduced risks of diabetic complications.

More than 60 years ago, **Elliott P. Joslin** was the first physician to speculate about the benefits of tight control. He theorized that diabetic complications could be minimized - even prevented in people with diabetes, if they kept their blood glucose as close to normal as possible. Unfortunately, diet control was impossible in Joslin's days because no quick efficient way to monitor blood glucose existed.

Few diseases have such widespread mixed effects on the body as diabetes. It virtually acts upon all tissues and organs in the body especially the pancreas, blood vessels, peripheral nerves, eyes and kidneys.

Major complications include :

(a) **Cardiovascular (heart) complications** including atherosclerosis,

(b) **Retinopathy (irreversible eye diseases),**

(c) **Nephropathy (severe damages to kidneys),**

(d) **Neuropathy (damage to the nervous system)** and many other severe complications.

More the hyperglycaemia, more the severity of complications.

Q.137. What is diabetic nephropathy?

Ans. Kidney disease (nephropathy) occurs when the blood distribution system (capillaries) of the kidney becomes leaky or plugged. **When it is plugged, filtration of urine gets hampered and blood continues to remain impure. When the capillaries become leaky, they will permit proteins and other major nutrients to escape from blood circulation thereby leading to the loss of essential components of blood. If diagnosed in time, it can prevent further damages by :**

(a) Controlling the causes of nephropathy (diabetes, hypertension or many others)

(b) Using certain drugs which can reduce the severity of damages (ACE inhibitors).

Q.138. What is ESRD?

Ans. Irrespective of the causes of nephropathy, in undiagnosed and/or uncontrolled diabetes, nephropathy will completely damage the entire functioning of the kidney and may result in severe complications which are known as ESRD (End Stage Renal Disease). As the very name suggests such situations are irreversible and the options would be either a kidney transplantation or dialysis and it is known that either of them can only delay the end.

Q.139. How diabetic nephropathy can be predicted?

Ans. The best indicator of nephropathy is the persistent presence of proteins in urine in quantities more than normal. Thus, for the last two decades it has been focussed to develop methods which can even detect the slightest increase in urinary albumin levels, leading to a concept of microalbuminuria.

Q.140. What is microalbuminuria?

Ans. Microalbuminuria (micro - very little, albuminuria-albumin in urine) Historically, diabetic nephropathy was recognized only when routine urine analysis revealed protein levels exceeding the detection levels of these assays i.e. 200-300 mg/dl. However, the sensitivity of such levels do not help in identifying any early stage of nephropathy though they were the only tests which signalled the onset of nephropathy. Hence, newer techniques are available for the detection of albumin in the smallest quantity i.e. even less than 20 mg/ml.

Q.141. How is microalbuminuria estimated?

Ans. Microalbuminuria should be estimated using techniques like RIA (radioimmunoassay - a nobel prize winning technology), CLIA (Chemiluminescence immunoassay) which are quantitative immunoassays having sensitivity as low as 0.25 mg/ml.

Q.142. What is c-peptide?

Ans. Pancreas synthesizes insulin through a precursor called proinsulin. In other words, proinsulin is a protein which gets cleaved into two different proteins called insulin and c-peptide.

$$\text{Proinsulin} \longrightarrow \text{Insulin} + \text{c-peptide}$$

C-peptide does not have any metabolic effect in human body. Insulin and c-peptide are synthesized in equal quantities and it is because insulin gets metabolized faster than c-peptide (half life of insulin is 5-10 minutes where as that of **c-peptide** is 30-40 minutes), the circulating level of c-peptide is higher.

Q.143. What is the utility of c-peptide test?

Ans. (a) Since c-peptide also originates from pancreatic cells, diabetologists use c-peptide measurements in conjunction with insulin levels **to assess the true pancreatic reserve.**

(b) C-peptide is used to **indirectly monitor insulin secretion** in the presence of anti-insulin antibodies (good number of **patients who are on insulin injections produce** autoantibodies to insulin) and help settle as an appropriate course of treatment; commercial preparation of insulin do not contain c-peptide.

Q.144. What are the after effects/complications of anxiety during venipunctures in an individual?

Ans. Even anxiety over venipunctures may generate enough epinephrine to produce an abnormal glucose tolerance test/blood sugar estimation. Coexisting illness, inadequate diet and lack of physical exercise also contribute to false positive tests.

Q.145. What is the most common endocrine disease of the day?

Ans. Diabetes mellitus.

Q.146. On which chromosome, the gene for the synthesis of Insulin is found to be located?

Ans. Chromosome No. 11.

Q.147. How many amino acids are found in human preproinsulin and what is its molecular weight?

Ans. 108 amino acids, M.W. is 11,500 daltons.

Q.148. How many amino acids are found in human proinsulin and what is its molecular weight?

Ans. 86 amino acids, M.W. is 9,390 daltons.

Q.149. How many amino acids are found in human insulin and what is its molecular weight?

Ans. 51 amino acids, M.W. is 5,808 daltons.

Q.150. In which concentration, insulin and C-peptide are produced?

Ans. Equimolar concentration.

Q.151. What is the biological activity of c-peptide?

Ans. Nil.

Q.152. What is the significance of the estimation of c-peptide in plasma?

Ans. Its estimation in the plasma serves as a useful index for the endogenous production of insulin.

Q.153. In which form, insulin is stored in the granules of the cytosol?

Ans. In complex form with zinc. In the β-cells, insulin (and also proinsulin) combines with zinc to form complexes.

Q.154. What is the normal fasting insulin concentration in plasma?

Ans. < 25 mIU/l (<174pmol/l).

Q.155. What is the half-life of insulin receptor?

Ans. 6-12 hours.

Q.156. What is the approximate number of receptors per cell in the mammals?

Ans. About 20,000

Q.157. What is the chemistry of insulin receptor?

Ans. It is a tetramer consisting of 4 subunits of two types and is designated as a_2 b_2. The subunits are in glycosylated form. They are held together by disulfide bridges. The a-subunit (M.W. 135,000) is extracellular and it contains insulin binding site. The b-subunit (M.W. 95,000) is a transmembrane protein which is activated by insulin. The cytoplasmic domain of b-subunit has tyrosine kinase activity.

Q.158 What are the various metabolic alterations in carbohydrate, lipid and protein metabolisms in diabetes mellitus?

Ans. These are as follows :

Metabolic alterations in DM

Carbohydrate metabolism	Lipid metabolism	Protein metabolism
Hyperglycaemia	Hyperlipemia	Catabolism of tissue protein ↑
Gluconeogenesis ↑	Lipoprotein lipase activity ↓	Protein synthesis ↓
Glycogenesis ↓	T G lipase activity ↑	Fatty liver possible
Glycolysis ↓	β-oxidation ↑	
Glycogenolysis ↑	Acetyl CoA ↑	
Glucose entry into cell ↓	Ketone bodies formation ↑	
	Cholesterol synthesis ↑	

Q.159. What do you understand by the words 'intermediary metabolism' and 'energy metabolism'?

Ans. The term intermediary metabolism is used for the entire range of catabolic and anabolic reactions, whereas energy metabolism is confined to the metabolic pathways concerned with the storage and liberation of energy.

Q.160. Name the enzymes catalyzing irreversible reactions of glycolysis.

Ans. (i) Hexokinase (glucokinase),
(ii) Phosphofructokinase, and
(iii) Pyruvate kinase

Q.161. What are the major differences between the enzymes hexokinase and glucokinase?

Ans. Differences between Hexokinase and Glucokinase

Sl. No.		Hexokinase	Glucokinase
1	Occurrence	Ubiquitous, i.e., found in all tissues	Found mainly in liver
2.	Affinity to substrate	High affinity	Low affinity

3.	Km value	Low km (about 0.01 mM) for substrates	High km (10 mM)for glucose
4.	V_{max}	Low	High
5.	Feedback inhibition	Feedback inhibited by glucose-6-phosphate	No direct feedback inhibition
6.	Induction by insulin	Not induced by insulin	Induced by insulin
7.	Specificity	Acts on all hexoses, i.e., glucose, fructose & mannose (catalyses the phosphorylation of all hexoses)	Acts on glucose only (catalyses the phosphorylation of glucose only)
8.	Capacity	Low	High
9.	Function, i.e., phosphorylation	Acts even when blood sugar level is low, glucose is phosphorylated, vis-a-vis utilised by the cells of the body.	Acts only when blood sugar level is high (more than 100 mg/dl), then, glucose is taken up for phosphorylation by the cells of the liver for the synthesis of glycogen **(glycogenesis).**

Q.162. What do you understand by Pasteur effect?

Ans. The inhibition of glycolysis by oxygen is referred to as Pasteur effect. This is due to the inhibition of the enzyme PFK by ATP and citrate (formed in the presence of oxygen).

Q.163. What is Rapport-Leubering cycle and its importance?

Ans. It is a supplementary pathway to glycolysis which operates in RBCs of men and other mammals. This cycle is mainly concerned with the synthesis of 2, 3 - diphosphoglycerate in the RBCs which facilitates the release of oxygen from oxyhaemoglobin in the tissues.

Q.164. What do you know about glycogenin?

Ans. It is a specific protein which can act as a primer (in the absence of glycogen primer) for the synthesis of glycogen. The hydroxyl group of the amino acid tyrosine of glycogenin is the site at which the initial glucose unit gets attached.

Q.165. What is the importance of uronic acid pathway?

Ans. Uronic acid (or glucuronic acid) pathway is an oxidative pathway of glucose which is concerned with the synthesis of so many important substances in the body, like :

(i) Glucuronic acid,
(ii) Pentoses, and
(iii) Ascorbic acid i.e., vitamin C (not in humans).

Q.166. What is sorbitol pathway?

Ans. Sorbitol (polyol) pathway basically involves the conversion of glucose to fructose via sorbitol. This pathway is related to glucose concentration and **remains higher in uncontrolled diabetic cases.** The pathological changes associated with diabetes mellitus like cataract formation, nephropathy, peripheral neuropathy, etc. are believed to be due to the accumulation of sorbitol.

Q.167. What is essential fructosuria?

Ans. The deficiency of enzyme fructokinase causes **'essential fructosuria'** which is an asymptomatic condition associated with the excretion of fructose in urine.

Q.168. What is hereditary fructose intolerance?

Ans. Deficiency of enzyme aldolase-B causes hereditary fructose intolerance that might lead to severe hypoglycemia, vomiting, jaundice, hepatic failure, etc.

Q.169. In how many hours half of the blood glucose is lost via glycolysis on standing?

Ans. 2-3 hours.

Q.170. Why blood glucose is lost on standing? Which chemical reaction takes place upon standing?

Ans. Due to glycolysis, as a result of which glucose gets converted to lactic acid upon standing. The reaction takes place as follows :

$$\underset{\text{glucose}}{C_6H_{12}O_6} \longrightarrow \underset{\text{lactic acid}}{2C_3H_6O_3}$$

Q.171. For how many days, the mixture of sodium fluoride and potassium oxalate can prevent glycolysis from taking place i.e., loss of glucose in the blood sample?

Ans. 2-3 days

Q.172. Name the glucose tolerance factor which increases sugar tolerance.

Ans. Chromium, Cr^{3+}

Q.173. What do you understand by the word insulicopenia?

Ans. It means pertaining to a decrease in the level of circulating insulin.

Q.174. Which type of hormone is Insulin?

Ans. Peptide

Q.175. What is the normal secretion of insulin per day?

Ans. Nearly 2 mg (50 units)

Q.176. What is lactose intolerance?

Ans. Some adults are unable to metabolize milk sugar, i.e., lactose and face gastrointestinal disturbances upon drinking milk. This condition when one is unable to tolerate milk sugar is called **lactose intolerance** or **hypolactasia.** This is most commonly caused due to the deficiency of enzyme **lactase** which breaks lactose into its constituents, i.e., glucose and galactose.

Q.177. What is the plus point of consuming milk sugar (lactose)?

Ans. Lactose is a food source of energy for microorganisms in the colon and they ferment it to lactic acid and also generate methane and hydrogen gases as well.

Q.178. Are there any side effect(s) of methane and hydrogen gases in the gut?

Ans. The gases so produced are responsible for :

(a) Distension of gut causing discomfort, and

(b) Flatulence

Q.179. Is there any side effect of the production of lactic acid (lactate) in the colon?

Ans. **Lactic acid**, thus, produced is osmotically active and draws water into the intestine, causing diarrhoea. If severe enough, the gases and diarrhoea hinder the absorption of other nutrients such as fat and protein. The simplest treatment is to avoid consumption of milk products (containing lactose).

Q.180. Name various rate limiting enzymes of various pathways/cycles of carbohydrate metabolism.

Ans.

Sl. No.	Pathway/Cycle	Name of the Enzyme
1.	Glycolysis	PFK-1
2.	Glycogenesis	Glycogen synthetase
3.	Glycogenolysis	Glycogenphosphorylase
4.	Gluconeogenesis	Fructose-1, 6-diphos-phatase
5.	HMP shunt	Glucose-6-phosphate dehydrogenase
6.	TCA Cycle	Isocitrate dehydrogenase

Q.181. Name the enzymes which are found deficient /missing in hereditary fructose intolerance (HFI), essential fructosuria and galactosaemia.

Ans. (i) Aldolase-B,

(ii) Fructokinase, and

(iii) Galactose-1-phosphate uridyl transferase, respectively.

Q.182. Name the glycogen storage diseases and their missing enzymes?

Ans.

Type	Glycogen storage disease (s)	Deficient enzyme (missing)
I	Von Gierke disease	Glucose-6-phosphatase
II	Pompe's disease	Acid maltase (Lysosomal)
III	Limit dextrinosis/ Forbes' disease or Cori disease	Debranching enzyme, i.e., Amylo-1,6-glucosidase
IV	Amylopectinosis or Andersen's disease	Branching enzyme, i.e., (Amylo-[1→4]→[1→6] transglucosidase)
V	McArdle's disease	Muscle phosphorylase
VI	Her's disease	Liver phosphorylase
VII	Tarui disease	Phosphofructokinase
VIII	–	Liver phosphorylase kinase

Q.183. What is the incidence of hereditary fructose intolerance (HFI)?

Ans. 1 in 20,000 live births

Q.184. What are the side effects of HFI?

Ans. Prolonged intake of fructose by infants with this defect leads to:

(i) Vomiting
(ii) Jaundice
(iii) Poor feeding
(iv) Hepatomegaly
(v) Hemorrhage
(vi) Hepatic failure, and
(vii) Eventually death

Q.185. What is the side effect of essential fructosuria?

Ans. Disease depends upon the intake of fructose and sucrose, it's asymptomatic and harmless and may go undiagnosed.

Q.186. What is the classification of diabetes mellitus?

Ans. It's as follows :-

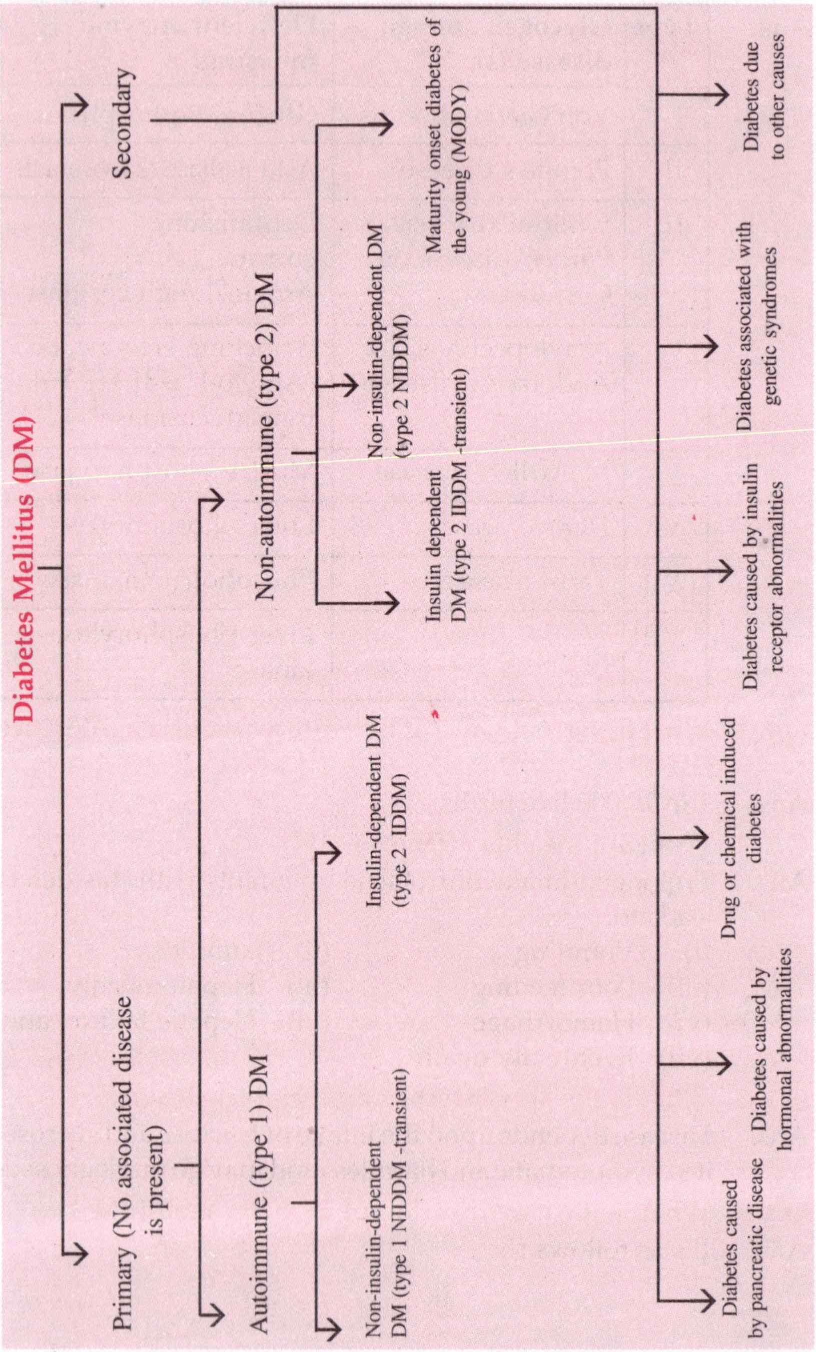
Diabetes Mellitus (DM)
Primary (No associated disease is present)
Secondary
Autoimmune (type 1) DM
Non-autoimmune (type 2) DM
Non-insulin-dependent DM (type 1 NIDDM -transient)
Insulin-dependent DM (type 2 IDDM)
Insulin dependent DM (type 2 IDDM -transient)
Non-insulin-dependent DM (type 2 NIDDM)
Maturity onset diabetes of the young (MODY)
Diabetes caused by pancreatic disease
Diabetes caused by hormonal abnormalities
Drug or chemical induced diabetes
Diabetes caused by insulin receptor abnormalities
Diabetes associated with genetic syndromes
Diabetes due to other causes

3

LIPIDS

Q.1. What are lipids?

Ans. They are esters of fatty acids which are characterized by their insolubility in water and solubility in fat solvents like ether, chloroform, benzene, CCl_4, etc.

Q.2. Name the fat depots of human body.

Ans. (i) Subcutaneous connective tissue
(ii) Intermuscular connective tissue
(ii) Omentum, etc.

Q.3. What is the classification of lipids?

Ans. They have been classified into three categories:

- (i) Simple lipids
  - Fat and oils
  - Waxes
- (ii) Compound or Conjugate lipids
  - Phospholipids
  - Glycolipids
  - Sulpholipids
  - Lipoproteins
- (iii) Derived lipids
  - Fatty acids
  - Alcohols
  - Hydrocarbons
  - Vitamin D
  - Vitamin E
  - Vitamin K

Q.4. What are fats?

Ans. They are esters of fatty acids with glycerol which are solid at room temperature.

Q.5. What are oils?

Ans. They are also esters of fatty acids with glycerol which are liquid at room temperature.

Q.6. What is the importance of lipids?

Ans. (i) They act as heat insulators

(ii) They are reservoirs of energy

(iii) They are constituents of cell membranes

(iv) They yield approximately 9 calories per gram which is more than twice than what is obtained from equivalent amount of carbohydrates and proteins

(v) They serve as vehicles for the fat soluble vitamins i.e. A, D, E and K

(vi) They provide essential fatty acids (EFA).

Q.7. Name the saturated fatty acids which are abundantly found in the fats.

Ans. (i) Palmitic acid i.e., $C_{15}H_{31}COOH$

(ii) Stearic acid i.e., $C_{17}H_{35}COOH$

Q.8. What is the full form of PUFA?

Ans. Poly Unsaturated Fatty Acids.

Q.9. Name 3 PUFA.

Ans. (i) Linoleic acid (ii) Linolenic acid

(iii) Arachidonic acid

Q.10. What are essential fatty acids (EFAs)?

Ans. Essential fatty acids are those which are not synthesized by the body and hence their supply through diet is necessary. They are also called polyunsaturated fatty acids. These include :

Sl. No.	Essential Fatty Acid	No. of double bonds	No. of carbon atoms
(i)	Linoleic acid $C_{17}H_{31}COOH$	$2,\Delta^{9,12}$	18
(ii)	Linolenic acid $C_{17}H_{29}COOH$	$3,\Delta^{9,12,15}$	18
(iii)	Arachidonic acid $C_{19}H_{31}COOH$	$4,\Delta^{5,8,11,14}$	20

Actually, since mammals can synthesize arachidonic acid and linolenic acid from *linoleic acid*, the latter i.e. *linoleic acid* only is essential in the real sense. The pathway would then appear as:

$$\text{linoleic} \xrightarrow{-2H} \text{linolenic} \xrightarrow{+C_2} \text{homo-linolenic} \xrightarrow{-2H} \text{arachidonic}$$

Q.11. What are the sources of EFA?

Ans. (i) Linseed oil (ii) Cottonseed oil
(iii) Soyabean oil (iv) Corn oil
(v) Peanut oil (vi) Egg-yolk
(vii) Rapeseed oil (viii) Fish-viscera, etc.

Q.12. What are the functions of essential fatty acids?

Ans. (i) They prevent deposition of cholesterol in the coronary arteries and other arteries as well by decreasing biosynthesis of cholesterol either from saturated fatty acids or non-fat sources.
(ii) They are the precursors of prostaglandins.

Q.13. Name five saturated fatty acids with their sources.

Ans. (i) Butyric acid - Butter
(ii) Caproic acid - Butter, coconut oil
(iii) Caprylic acid - Butter, coconut oil
(iv) Capric acid - Butter, coconut oil
(v) Palmitic acid - Most vegetables and animal fats

Q.14. Name two unsaturated fatty acids with one double bond in their structure.

Ans. (i) Palmitoleic acid (ii) Oleic acid

Q.15. Name one unsaturated fatty acid with two double bonds in its structure.

Ans. Linoleic acid.

Q.16. Name one unsaturated fatty acid with three double bonds in its structure.

Ans. Linolenic acid.

Q.17. Name one unsaturated fatty acid with four double bonds in its structure.

Ans. Arachidonic acid.

Q.18. What is the composition of lecithins?

Ans. Lecithins contain:
(i) Glycerol (ii) Fatty acids
(iii) Phosphoric acid and (iv) Choline

Q.19. What is the composition of cephalins?

Ans. Cephalins contain :

(i) Glycerol (ii) Fatty acids
(iii) Phosphoric acid, and (iv) Ethanolamine

Q.20. Where is lecithinase A found and what is its action on lecithin molecule?

Ans. It's found in the venoms of certain snakes like cobra, vipers etc., poisons of scorpions and bees and various mammalian tissues. It specifically hydrolyzes of the fatty acid from the lecithin molecule in order to form lysolecithin which is a very powerful hemolytic agent.

Q.21. What are cerebrosides?

Ans. These are lipids which contain:
(i) Carbohydrate (galactose or glucose)
(ii) One fatty acid, and (iii) Sphingosine

Q.22. What is saponification?

Ans. Hydrolysis of fat by an alkali is called saponification.

Q.23. What is saponification number?

Ans. Saponification number is defined as the milligrams of KOH required to saponify 1 gm of fat.

Q.24. What does the saponification number of a fat indicate?

Ans. Saponification number of a fat gives an idea about the average chain length of the fatty acids present in the fat. Higher the saponification number, the shorter (or smaller) will be the chain length of the fatty acid and vice versa.

Q.25. What is iodine number?

Ans. Iodine number is defined as the grams of iodine absorbed by 100g of fat.

Q.26. What does the iodine number indicate?

Ans. Iodine number indicates the degree of unsaturation of the fat. Higher the iodine number, more is the degree of unsaturation of the fat.

Q.27. What are antioxidants?

Ans. Antioxidants are substances that prevent rancidity. They also control and reduce lipid peroxidation both in nature and humans.

Q.28. What is rancidity of fats?

Ans. Rancidity of fats is a chemical change due to ageing which results in the unpleasant odour and taste of the fat on storage when they are exposed to light, heat and moisture etc.

Q. 29. Which vitamin prevents rancidity?

Ans. Vitamin E

Q.30. What are steroids?

Ans. Substances possessing cyclopenteno perhydrophenanthrene nucleus are called steroids, structure is as shown below :

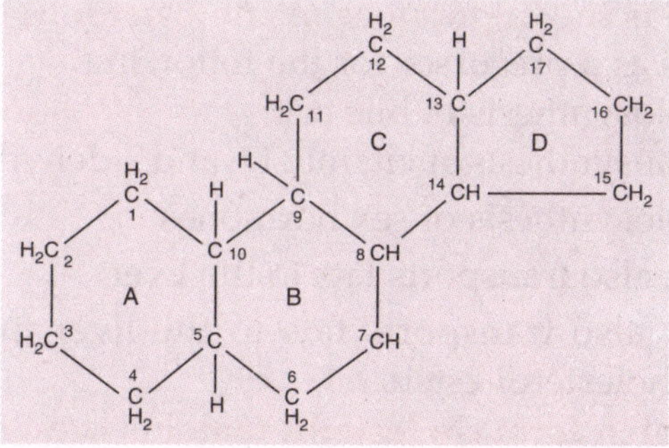

Q.31. What is the molecular formula of cholesterol?

Ans. $C_{27}H_{45}OH$

Q.32. Can you name other antioxidants?

Ans. (i) Lipid soluble :

(a) Vitamin E (b) β-carotene

(ii) Water soluble :

(a) Vitamin C (b) Urates

(iii) Preventive antioxidants

(a) Catalases (b) EDTA

(c) Hydroquinone

(iv) Chain breaking antioxidants

(a) Phenols (b) Superoxide dismutase

Q.33. Give the structure of cholesterol.

Ans.

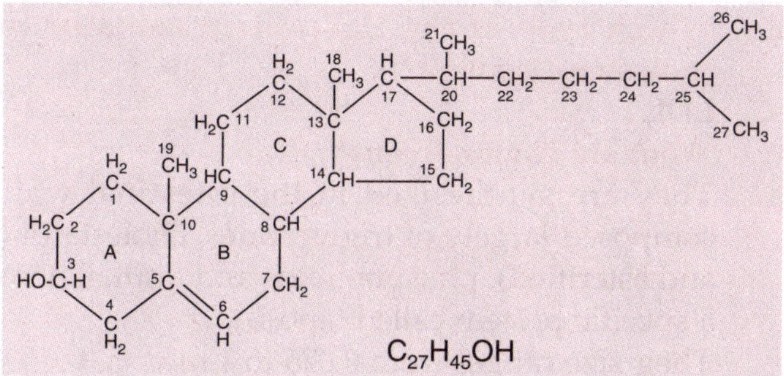

$C_{27}H_{45}OH$

Q.34. What is the full form of CPP nucleus?

Ans. Cyclopenteno perhydro phenanthrene

Q.35. What are the tests by which cholesterol is detected?

Ans. (i) Liebermann-Burchard reaction

(ii) Salkowski test

Q.36. What is the importance of cholesterol in the body?

Ans. It acts as a precursor for the following:

(a) Biosynthesis of bile acids

(b) Biosynthesis of vitamin D_3 and 7-dehydrocholesterol

(c) Biosynthesis of sex hormones

(d) It also transports fats to the liver

(e) It also transports fats to the liver in the form of cholesterol esters.

Q.37. In which form cholesterol remains present in blood?

Ans. (i) Free cholesterol (25-35% of the total cholesterol)

(ii) Esterified cholesterol (65-75% of the total cholesterol).

Q.38. What are lipotropic factors? Give examples.

Ans Those substances which prevent liver from becoming fatty are known as lipotropic factors. Examples are :

(i) Choline (ii) Betaine

(iii) Methionine (iv) Inositol, etc.

Q.39. Mention the major groups of lipoproteins which are physiologically and diagnostically important.

Ans. (i) Very low density lipoproteins (VLDL), i.e. pre-β-lipoproteins

(ii) Low density lipoproteins (LDL), i.e. β-lipoproteins

(iii) High density lipoproteins (HDL_1, HDL_2 and HDL_3), i.e. α-lipoproteins.

Q.40. Which type of the lipoprotein contains maximum cholesterol content?

Ans. LDL

Q.41. What are chylomicrons?

Ans. They are synthesized in the intestinal wall and are composed largely of triglycerides, cholesterol (both free and esterified), phospholipids and a small percentage of a specific protein called 'apo-B_{48}'.

Their size ranges from 0.075 to 1 mμ.

Q.42. What are lipoproteins?

Ans. The combination of lipid with protein is called lipoprotein.

Q.43. What are apolipoproteins i.e. apoproteins?

Ans. The protein component of plasma lipoproteins is called apolipoprotein.

Apoproteins are of five types i.e., A, B, C, D and E

Q.44. What are bile salts?

Ans. They are sodium and potassium salts of glycocholates and taurocholates i.e.

(i) Sodium glycocholate
(ii) Potassium glycocholate
(iii) Sodium taurocholate
(iv) Potassium taurocholate

Q.45. What are the main functions of bile salts?

Ans. (i) As powerful emulsifying agents
(ii) Lowering of surface tension
(iii) They accelerate the action of enzyme pancreatic lipase
(iv) They keep cholesterol in solution
(v) They help in the absorption of fat soluble vitamins i.e., A, D, E and K.

Q.46 What is the classification of antioxidants?

Ans. (i) Lipid soluble :
(a) Vitamin E (b) β-carotene
(ii) Water soluble :
(a) Vitamin C (b) Urates
(iii) Preventive antioxidants
(a) Catalases (b) EDTA
(c) Hydroquinone
(iv) Chain breaking antioxidants
(a) Phenols (b) Superoxide dismutase.

4

Lipid Metabolism

Q.1. What is the main site of lipid metabolism?

Ans. Liver

Q.2. What is the percentage of lipid in a normal liver?

Ans. 5%

Q.3. What is the maximum percentage of lipid in 'fatty liver disease' (FLD) or steatosis hepatitis?

Ans. **30-40%,** this disease is reversible, main causes are alcohol intake & obesity or metabolic syndromes (diabetes, hypertension & dyslipidemia).

Q.4. Name the ketone bodies i.e. acetone bodies.

Ans. (i) Acetoacetic acid
(ii) β-hydroxybutyric acid and
(iii) Acetone

Q.5. By which qualitative test, ketone bodies are detected in urine?

Ans. Rothera's test

Q.6. What is ketogenesis? What are its precursors?

Ans. The phenomenon of the formation of ketone bodies is called as ketogenesis, its precursors include:

(i) Acetyl coenzyme A
(ii) Pyruvate
(iii) Acetic acid
(iv) Leucine
(v) Phenylalanine, etc.

Q. 7. What is ketosis? When does it take place?

Ans. When an excessive amount of fat is catabolized, ketone bodies are formed in massive quantity, this condition is known as **Ketosis** in which one finds raised level of **Ketone Bodies** in blood **(Ketonaemia)** and detectable appreciable amount of **Ketone Bodies** in urine **(Ketonuria).** Ketosis can occur :

(i) In a person undergoing a complete fast, where there are insufficient carbohydrates and excess fats in the diet, and

(ii) In **severe diabetes mellitus**. The disproportionate metabolism of lipids in diabetics is the cause of overproduction of **Ketone Bodies.**

Q.8. What happens when increased production of Ketone Bodies takes place as in severe diabetes mellitus?

Ans. It results in the depletion of the alkali reserve, causing acidosis.

Q.9. Where does the oxidation of fatty acids take place in the cell?

Ans. Mitochondria

Q.10. A fatty acid is degraded step by step by the sequential removal of how many carbon units?

Ans. Two

Q.11. Can liver utilize 'ketone bodies'? If not, why?

Ans. Liver cannot utilize ketone bodies because of the fact that the activating enzyme required for the utilization of ketone bodies is found to be absent in the liver.

Q.12. What is ketoacidosis?

Ans. When ketosis is severe, the patient's breath has a characteristic smell like acetone which is easily recognisable. Acetoacetic acid and β-hydroxybutyric acid are produced faster than they can be metabolized as a result of which these acids accumulate causing decrease in the pH of blood, a condition known as academia or ketoacidosis takes place which eventually gives rise to hyperventilation (air hunger).

Q.13. Are ketone bodies normal end products of fatty acid oxidation in the liver?

Ans. Yes, but in small amount.

Q.14. What is the normal level of ketone bodies in the blood?

Ans. It is upto 3 mg%.

Q.15. What is the outcome of the hydrolysis of triacylglycerol (triglyceride)?

Ans. Fatty acids are stored in the adipose tissue in the form of triacylglycerol which are mainly oxidized for energy purpose.

Mobilization of the stored fat requires hydrolytic release of the fatty acids and glycerol from TAG as per following scheme. The enzyme called hormone - sensitive lipase, which removes fatty acids from carbon -1 and/or 3 of a TAG, initiates this process. Additional lipases which are specific for DAGs and monoacylglycerols (MAGs) remove the remaining fatty acids.

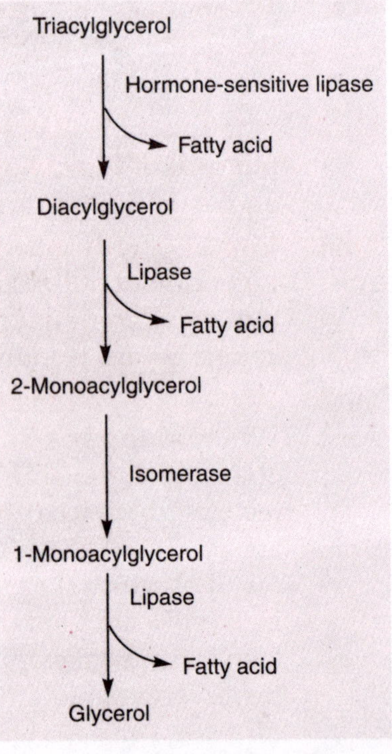

Fig. Breakdown of TAG

Q.16. What is the concentration of ketone bodies in the blood in diabetics?

Ans. It may be as much as 300-400 mg% or even more.

Q.17. What is the normal daily excretion of ketone bodies in the urine?

Ans. Upto 50 mg.

Q.18. What is the daily excretion of ketone bodies in the urine of diabetics?

Ans. 10-50 grams per litre

Q.19. What is the nature of ketone bodies?

Ans. Acidic

Q.20. What is the main site of the production of ketone bodies?

Ans. Liver

Q.21. Name the tissues which prefer ketone bodies for utilization.

Ans. Extrahepatic tissues prefer ketone bodies for utilization because they possess the activating enzymes.

Q.22. How are the ketone bodies formed?

Ans. These are formed as intermediate breakdown products of fat metabolism. If carbohydrate metabolism is defective, more lipid is broken down for energy purposes, hence more of the ketone bodies are formed.

Q.23. Name the regulatory enzyme of cholesterol biosynthesis.

Ans. β–hydroxy–β–methyl glutaryl CoA **(HMG CoA).**

Q.24. What are the plus points of catabolism of cholesterol?

Ans. It is the mother of so many valuable substances, i.e.

(i) Bile acids
(ii) Androgenic hormones (testosterone, etc.)
(iii) Estrogenic hormones (estradiol and estrone etc.)
(iv) Glucocorticoid hormones (cortisol, cortisone, etc.)
(v) Mineralocorticoid hormones (aldosterone, etc.).

Q.25. What are the sites of cholesterol biosynthesis?

Ans. (i) Liver
(ii) Skin, and
(iii) Adrenal cortical tissue

Q.26. What is the precursor of cholesterol biosynthesis?

Ans. Acetyl CoA (2 molecules)

Q.27. Give a short diagram to show the biosynthesis of cholesterol.

Ans. 2 moles of Acetyl CoA ⟶ Acetoacetyl CoA ⟶ Mevalonic acid ⟶ Squalene ⟶ Lanosterol ⟶ Desmosterol ⟶ Cholesterol

Q.28. Where are the enzymes of cholesterol biosynthesis found in the cell?

Ans. Endoplasmic reticulum

Q.29. What type of chemical is carnitine?

Ans. It is γ-trimethyl ammonium β-hydroxy-butyrate.

Q.30. What is the role of carnitine?

Ans. It plays a very important role as it acts as a **carrier of fatty acids** which are transported across the inner membrane of the mitochondria to the matrix in the cytosol for oxidation purposes.

Q.31. By which mechanisms fatty acids are oxidized in our system and which is the main mechanism?

Ans. (i) α-oxidation (ii) β-oxidation, and (iii) ω-oxidation

β-oxidation is the main mechanism (principal pathway).

Q.32. What is the other name of β-oxidation theory?

Ans. Knoop's β-oxidation theory.

Q.33. Where does β-oxidation takes place?

Ans. Mitochondria

Q.34. How many molecules of ATP are generated by the complete oxidation (β-oxidation + TCA cycle) of one molecule of palmitic acid (sixteen carbon fatty acid)?

Ans. 106 [($7FADH_2 \times 1.5$ ATP = 10.5 ATP; 7NADH x 2.5 ATP = 17.5 ATP; i.e., total 10.5 + 17.5 = 28 ATP) + 8 Acetyl CoA forming 80 ATP; grand total = 28 + 80 ATP = 108 - 2 ATP = 106 ATP].

Q.35. How many molecules of ATP are generated by the complete oxidation (β-oxidation + TCA cycle) of one molecule of stearic acid (eighteen carbon fatty acid)?

Ans. 121 (Stearic acid contains 18 carbon atoms. There are 8 turns of β-oxidation and 9 molecules of acetyl CoA are formed. Acetyl CoA enters TCA cycle. One mole of ATP is used for the activation of stearic acid.

Hence, the total ATP = (8 x 4) + (9 x 10) - 1 = 121 [(8$FADH_2$ x 1.5 ATP = 12 ATP; 8NADH + 2.5 ATP = 20 ATP, total 12 + 20 = 32 ATP) + 9Acetyl CoA forming 90 ATP; grand total = 122 -1 ATP = 121 ATP]

Q.36. What is β-oxidation?

Ans. In this type, oxidation takes place at the β-carbon atom and the β-carbon is oxidized to carboxyl group i.e., COOH.

Q.37. Name the simplest fatty acid.

Ans. **Acetic acid** is the simplest fatty acid with an even number of carbon atoms. It undergoes activation of acetyl CoA and mixes with the acetyl CoA pool of the body.

Q.38. How does oxidation of fatty acids with odd number of carbon atoms take place?

Ans.

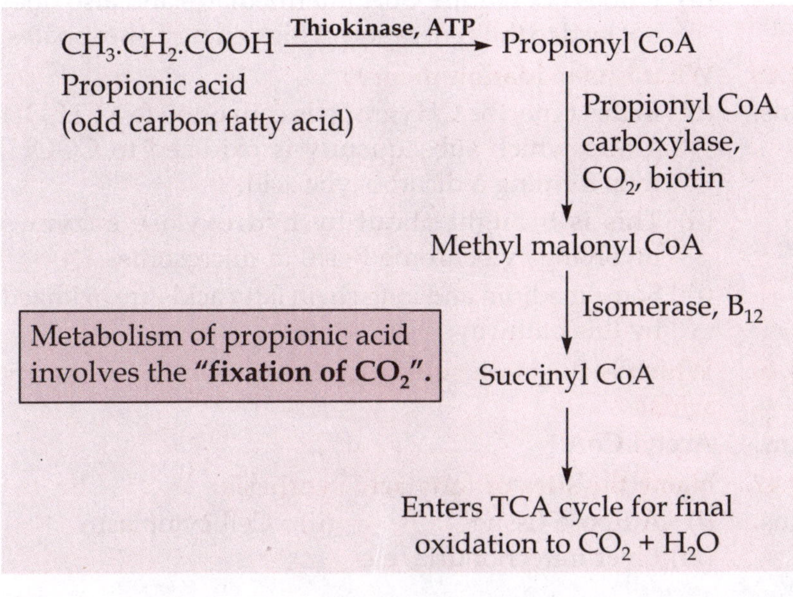

Q.39. Name glycogenic fatty acids.

Ans. (i) Acetic acid (ii) Propionic acid, etc.

Q.40. Name the chief fat-depots of the body.

Ans. (i) Subcutaneous fatty tissue
(ii) Retroperitoneal fatty tissue, and
(iii) Inter-muscular fatty tissue.

Q.41. What is β-oxidation theory of fatty acids?

Ans. Fatty acid first gets combined with coenzyme A to form acyl-CoA. After β-oxidation, the 2-C fragment splits off as acetyl CoA. This process is repeated until all the fatty acids are converted into acetyl CoA molecules.

Q.42. What happens to these acetyl CoA molecules?

Ans. These are oxidized to CO_2 and H_2O via TCA cycle releasing energy in the form of ATP.

Q.43. How many moles of ATP are formed by one turn of β-oxidation?

Ans. Five

Q.44. What is α-oxidation theory?

Ans. (i) In this type, removal of one carbon at a time occurs from the carboxyl end of the molecule.
(ii) It does not require CoA intermediates and also does not lead to the generation of high energy phosphates.

Q.45. What is ω-oxidation theory?

Ans. (i) In this type, the CH_3 group is converted to a CH_2OH group which subsequently is oxidized to COOH, thus forming a dicarboxylic acid.
(ii) This is brought about by hydroxylase enzymes involving cytochrome P-450 in microsomes.
(iii) Some medium and long chain fatty acids are oxidized by this pathway.

Q.46. Which is the main substance for the synthesis of fatty acids?

Ans. Acetyl CoA

Q.47. Name the sites of fatty acid synthesis.

Ans. (i) Adipose tissue (ii) Cell cytoplasm
(iii) Liver mitochondria, etc.

Q.48. What about the fate of fatty acid synthesis in diabetes mellitus?

Ans. It almost stops. In diabetes mellitus, there is not only a reduced supply of acetyl CoA from pyruvate because of decreased carbohydrate metabolism but there is also a reduced supply of NADPH.

Q.49. What are lipotropic factors, name them?

Ans. Those substances which prevent liver from becoming fatty by the deposition of triglycerides are known as **lipotropic factors**. Which include :

(i) Choline,
(ii) Betaine,
(iii) Methionine,
(iv) Inositol, and
(v) Lipocaic

These are required for the conversion of triglycerides to phospholipids, and thus, help in the normal transport and utilization of lipids, especially in the liver.

Q.50. Which nucleotides play an important role in lipid synthesis?

Ans. Cytidine nucleotides

Q.51. What is a fatty liver?

Ans. Significant accumulation of triglycerides in the liver gives rise to fatty liver (more than 5%).

Q.52. Name the storage sites of lipid?

Ans. (i) Subcutaneous connective tissue
(ii) Intermuscular connective tissue
(iii) Omentum
(iv) Perirenal fat depots, and
(v) Genital fat.

Q.53. What is the relationship between polyunsaturated fatty acids and the cholesterol?

Ans. Polyunsaturated fatty acids have got a tendency to lower the plasma cholesterol level.

Q.54. What are the various pathways by which acetyl CoA is utilized?

Ans. (i) Acetyl CoA gives rise to CO_2 and H_2O by TCA cycle
(ii) Acetyl CoA is utilized in the synthesis of fatty acids via malonyl CoA
(iii) Acetyl CoA gives rise to the synthesis of cholesterol
(iv) It also gives rise to acetoacetic acid i.e., ketone bodies
(v) It also undergoes acetylation reactions.

Q.55. What are the sources of acetyl CoA?

Ans. (i) Carbohydrate metabolism i.e., glycolysis
(ii) Fat metabolism i.e., β-oxidation of fatty acids
(iii) Protein metabolism i.e., transamination.

Q.56. What is Gaucher's disease?

Ans. It is a rare hereditary disease of lipid metabolism in which large amounts of cerebrosides accumulate in the liver and spleen. Enzyme deficient/missing is **β-glucosidase**. Liver and spleen become enlarged. Erosion of long bones also takes place and mental retardation in infants.

Q.57. What is Niemann–Pick disease?

Ans. It is a rare hereditary disease of lipid metabolism in which large amounts of **sphingomyelin** accumulate in the liver and brain. Enzyme deficient/missing is **sphingomyelinase**. Mental retardation takes place and liver and spleen become enlarged.

Q.58. What is Tay-Sachs disease?

Ans. It is also a rare hereditary disease of lipid metabolism in which large amounts of **gangliosides** accumulate in the brain. Enzyme deficient/missing in this disorder is **hexosaminidase A**. Mental retardation, blindness and muscular weakness take place.

Q.59. Name four diseases of lipid metabolism (lipidoses).

Ans. (i) Gaucher's disease (ii) Niemann-Pick disease
(iii) Tay-Sachs disease (iv) Fabry's disease.

Q.60. Which type of lipoprotein contains maximum cholesterol?

Ans. LDL

Q.61. For what increased concentration of cholesterol in blood (hypercholesterolaemia) is responsible?

Ans. Degenerative changes in the arterial walls (**atherosclerosis**).

Q.62 What chemically is HDL-cholesterol?

Ans. High density lipoproteins (HDL) contain particles of different densities including lipid and highest concentration of proteins.

It includes :

(i) Free and esterified cholesterol,
(ii) Triglycerides,
(iii) Phospholipids, and
(iv) Apoproteins A, C and E

Q.63 To which type of ailments, decreased level of HDL-cholesterol may be correlated?

Ans. There exists an inverse relationship between HDL cholesterol and coronary heart diseases. Low concentration i.e. **below 30 mg/dl is one of the risk factors for cardiac ailments.**

Q.64 What is the principle for the estimation of HDL-cholesterol?

Ans. Chylomicrons, LDL and VLDL (low and very low density lipoproteins) are precipitated from serum by phosphotungstate in the presence of divalent cations such as magnesium as shown below: HDL cholesterol remains unaffected in the supernatant and is estimated using cholesterol reagent.

$$\text{Serum/plasma} \xrightarrow[\text{Mg}^{2+}]{\text{Phosphotungstate}} \underset{\text{(supernatant)}}{\text{HDL}} + \underset{\text{(precipitate)}}{(\text{LDL} + \text{VLDL})}$$

Q.65 What is the normal level of HDL-cholesterol in males and females?

Ans. Males : 30-63 mg/dl
Females : 35-75 mg/dl

Q.66 What is the clinical significance of the measurement of serum cholesterol?

Ans. Its measurement in blood is useful in the evaluation of the risk of the coronary arterial occlusion, atherosclerosis, myocardial infarction, intestinal absorption, thyroid function and adrenal disease.

Q.67 In which disorders, high values of cholesterol are found.

Ans. (i) Primary hyperlipoproteinaemias
(ii) Nephrotic syndrome
(iii) Myxoedema
(iv) Obstructive jaundice, and
(v) Diabetes mellitus

Q.68 In which disorders, low values of cholesterol are found?

Ans. (i) Anemias
(ii) Haemolytic jaundice
(iii) Malabsorption syndrome
(iv) Severe malnutrition
(v) Acute infections, etc.

Q.69 In which disorders, very low values of cholesterol are found?

Ans. (i) Abetalipoproteinaemia, and to a lesser degree in
(ii) Familial hypobetalipoproteinaemias

Q.70 What happens when cholesterol esterase (CE) acts upon cholesterol ester?

Ans. $\text{Cholesterol ester} \xrightarrow{\text{CE}} \text{cholesterol + fatty acid}$

Q.71 What happens when cholesterol oxidase(CHOD) acts upon cholesterol?

Ans. $\text{Cholesterol} + O_2 \xrightarrow{\text{CHOD}} \text{cholest–4–en–3–one} + H_2O_2$

Q.72. What is the principle of enzymatic estimation of serum triglycerides?

Ans. It's as follows :

(i) $\text{Triglycerides} + H_2O \xrightarrow{\text{Lipase}} \text{Glycerol + free fatty acids}$

(ii) $\text{Glycerol + ATP} \xrightarrow{\text{GK}} \text{Glycerol-3-phosphate + ADP}$

(iii) $\text{Glycerol-3-phosphate} + O_2 \xrightarrow{\text{GPO}} \text{DAP} + H_2O_2$

(iv) $H_2O_2\text{+4AAP+3,5DHBS} \xrightarrow{\text{Peroxidase}} \underset{\text{(dye)}}{\text{Quinoneimine}} + 2H_2O$

Where,

GK = Glycerol kinase
GPO = Glycerol phosphate oxidase
DAP = Dihydroxyacetone phosphate
4–AAP = 4–Aminoantipyrine

DHBS = 3, 5—Dichloro—2—hydroxybenzene sulfonate.
The intensity of chromogen (Quinoneimine) formed is proportional to the triglycerides concentration.

Q.73. What is the equivalent concentration of 200 mg/dl in terms of mmol/L?

Ans. 5.2 mmol/L

Q.74. What does cause hepatic carnitine palmitoyltransferase deficiency cause?

Ans. It results in hypoglycaemia and low plasma ketone bodies.

Q.75. Which syndromes are caused due to the deficiency of enzyme muscle carnitine palmitoyltransferase?

Ans. It leads to impaired fatty acid oxidation that results in recurrent muscle weakness and myoglobinuria.

Q.76. What is Jamaican Vomiting Sickness?

Ans. It is caused by eating the unripe fruits of the Abee tree, which contains a toxin, called **hypoglycin,** that inactivates acyl-CoA dehydrogenase, inhibiting β-oxidation and causing hypoglycaemia.

Q.77. What is Refsum's disease?

Ans. Genetic deficiency of enzyme **α-hydroxylase (a monooxygenase)** results in an increase in the concentration of phytanic acid in blood and other tissues. This, in turn, leads to a neurological disorder called as **Refsum's disease**.

Q.78. What is Zellweger's (cerebrohepatorenal) syndrome?

Ans. It occurs in individuals with a rare inherited absence of peroxisomes in all the tissues in which polyenoic acids having carbon atoms ranging from C_{26} to C_{38} accumulate in brain tissue owing to inability to oxidize fatty acids of long-chain length in peroxisomes.

Q.79. Which type of lipoprotein contains maximum cholesterol?

Ans. LDL

Q.80. Approximately after how many hours blood triglycerides level reaches to a maximum postprandially?

Ans. 4-6 hours

Q.81. Related to which diseases, elevated levels of both cholesterol and triglycerides in blood have been identified as risk factors.

Ans. Coronary heart disease (atherosclerotic disease), hyperlipidemias, etc.

Q.82. What are the products formed when lipases act upon triglycerides?

Ans. Glycerol and fatty acids.

Q.83. What are the products formed when glycerokinase (GK) acts upon glycerol in the presence of ATP?

Ans. Glycerol phosphate and ADP

Q.84. Name ω 3,6 & 9 fatty acids.

Ans. (a) ω 3 fatty acid is **Linolenic acid** (18:3; 9,12,15 meaning chain length of 18 carbon atoms with three double bonds at carbon atom numbers 9,12 & 15)

(b) ω 6 fatty acids are **Linoleic acid** (18:2; 9,12) and **Arachidonic acid** (20:4; 5,8, 11, 14)

(c) ω 9 fatty acid is **Oleic acid** (18:1; 9)

(for instance ω 9 represents the double bond position (9 and 10) from the ω end). Naturally occurring unsaturated fatty acids belong to ω 9, ω 6 and ω 3 series.

Q.85. Why the intake of vitamin-E and omega-3 fatty acids essential?

Ans. (i) Vitamin-E is a powerful antioxidant, therefore essential.

(ii) Omega-3 fatty acids essential because of their thrombotic tendency.

(iii) Both improve various metabolic and vascular functions.

Q.86. Name some tissues which can not oxidize fatty acids for energy purpose.

Ans. (i) Brain, (ii) RBCs, and

(iii) Adrenal medulla

Q.87. What do you know about the regulation of hormone sensitive triacylglycerol lipase?

Ans. Hormone sensitive triacylglycerol (TG) lipase remains present in an inactive form 'b' and gets activated (phosphorylated) by a cyclic AMP dependent protein kinase to lipase 'a' which is an active form. Several hormones like epinephrine, norepinephrine, thyroxine, glucagon, etc. increase cAMP level and therefore, the activity of lipase causing increased lipolysis. However, the hormone insulin decreases cAMP level and thus inhibits lipolysis.

Q.88. What is sudden infant death syndrome (SIDS) or Reye's syndrome?

Ans. This syndrome is an unexpected death of healthy infants, usually in overnight, the exact cause of which is not yet very well understood. **It is now estimated that at least 10% of SIDS (Reye's syndrome) is due to the deficiency of the enzyme medium chain fatty acyl CoA dehydrogenase,** which, in turn, reduces fatty acid oxidation. Features of the disease include vomiting, lethargy and coma. Symptoms appear after more than 12 hours of fast and are more complicated on prolonged starvation, usually within 2 years of life. Treatment includes a carbohydrate rich diet.

Q.89. How are odd chain fatty acids oxidized?

Ans. β–oxidation of saturated fatty acids containing odd number of carbon atoms is similar to that of fatty acids with even carbons. The only difference is that in the last and final β–oxidation cycle, a 3–carbon fragment namely propionyl CoA is liberated (in place of acetyl CoA for even carbon fatty acids).

Q.90. What is the role of peroxisomes in fatty acid oxidation?

Ans. β–oxidation of fatty acids occurs in a modified form in peroxisomes without the generation of ATP (only heat is liberated). The reducing equivalents do not pass through ETC. Oxidation of fatty acids in peroxisomes is induced by high fat diet and administration of hypolipidemic drugs (e.g., clofibrate, lovastatin, etc).

Q.91. What is the first reaction in fatty acid synthesis?

Ans. Acetyl CoA is carboxylated to malonyl CoA by a biotin dependent enzyme called as acetyl CoA carboxylase which is a regulatory enzyme in fatty acid biosynthesis.

Q.92. Name the regulatory enzyme and other factors of fatty acid biosynthesis?

Ans. Its synthesis is regulated by the **enzyme acetyl CoA carboxylase (ACC)**, hormones (insulin hormone promotes whereas glucagon inhibits) and dietary manipulation (fasting or high fat diet decrease). In addition, the availability of NADPH (mostly generated in HMP pathway) also influences fatty acids synthesis.

Q.93. How is triacylglycerol synthesized?

Ans. Fatty acids and glycerol are activated and then by a series of reactions get converted to triacylglycerol (fat). Its synthesis mainly occurs in the liver and adipose tissue.

Q.94. How is cholesterol degraded?

Ans. Cholesterol is converted to bile acids (glycocholic acid, taurocholic acid). Cholesterol serves as a precursor for the synthesis of steroid hormones (cortisol, estradiol, progesterone), vitamin D, coprostanol and cholestanol. The latter two are the fecal sterols.

Q.95. What is cholelithiasis?

Ans. Cholelithiasis **(cholesterol gallstone disease)** is characterized by the deposition of cholesterol crystals in the gall bladder, this may occur due to the deficiency of bile salts or their defective absorption from the intestine, impairment in liver function, etc.

Q.96. What is LCAT and its importance?

Ans. Lecithin–cholesterol acyltransferase is found in plasma. Its activity remains associated with apo A1 of HDL and catalyses the transfer of a fatty acid from lecithin to cholesterol to produce cholesterol ester. In this way, cholesterol from the peripheral tissues is transported to the liver for degradation and excretion.

Q.97. What is hypercholesterolemia?

Ans. Increase in the normal level of cholesterol **(150-200 mg/dl)** is referred to as hypercholesterolemia which is observed in :

(i) Diabetes mellitus,
(ii) Obstructive jaundice,
(iii) Hypothyroidism, and
(iv) Nephrotic syndrome

Hypercholesterolemia is also found to be associated with atherosclerosis and coronary heart disease.

Q.98. What are lipoproteins?

Ans. These are molecular complexes which consist of lipids and proteins (conjugated protein). These function as transport vehicles (transporters) for lipids in blood plasma. There are 5 major classes of lipoproteins, i.e., chylomicrons, VLDL, LDL, HDL and free fatty acids–albumin.

Q.99. How are plasma lipoproteins separated from each other?

Ans. By electrophoresis.

Q.100. What are apolipoproteins or apoproteins?

Ans. These are the structural protein components of lipoproteins and remain closely involved in the metabolism of lipoproteins. Various apolipoproteins are divided into different classes from A to H. Most of the classes have subclasses like apo A-I, apo A-II, apo B-100 and apo B-48.

Q.101. What do you know about lipoprotein lipase?

Ans. This enzyme hydrolyzes a portion of the triacylglycerols present in chylomicrons and VLDL to liberate free fatty acids and glycerol. This enzyme is found in the capillary walls of adipose tissue, cardiac and skeletal muscles, etc.

Q.102. What are LDL receptors?

Ans. These are glycoproteins on the cell membrane. The shape of the receptor pits is stabilized by a protein known as clathrin. A defect in LDL receptors results in the elevation of plasma LDL, and hence plasma cholesterol. Deficiency of LDL receptors is observed in type IIa hyperbetalipoproteinemia which is associated with a very high risk of atherosclerosis.

Q.103. What do you know about hyperlipoproteinemias?

Ans. Elevation in one or more of the lipoproteins fractions is called as hyperlipoproteinemias or hyperlipidemias, the most acceptable classification of which is based on electrophoresis as type I, IIa, IIb, III, IV and V.

Q.104. What do you know about abetalipoproteinemia?

Ans. **It is a rare disorder due to a defect in the synthesis of apoprotein B which is characterized by a total absence of LDL in plasma.** This disorder is found to be associated with decreased absorption of fat and fat soluble vitamins. In this disorder retardation in physical growth and mental level are commonly observed.

Q.105. What is Tangier disease?

Ans. Familial alpha-lipoprotein deficiency is called as Tangier disease which is characterized by a total absence of HDL, adversely affecting the reverse transport of cholesterol resulting in the deposition of cholesterol esters in the tissues.

Q.106. What is obesity?

Ans. It is an abnormal increase in the body weight on account of excessive fat accumulation. Men and women are considered to be obese if their weight exceeds more than 20% and 25% of body weight respectively. **It is basically a disorder of excess calorie intake i.e. overeating.**

Q.107. What do you understand by anorexia nervosa?

Ans. By this word, we mean total loss of appetite. This is more a psychiatric problem, mostly seen in females in the age group of 10-30 years.

Q.108. What is the relation between high density lipoproteins (HDL) and coronary heart disease?

Ans. The elevated levels of plasma HDL are correlated with low incidence of cardiovascular disorders. Females have been reported to have higher plasma HDL and are less prone to heart disorders. **This has been attributed to estrogens in them.**

Q.109. What do you know about lipoprotein 'a'?

Ans. It is almost identical to LDL in structure and has a tendency to inhibit fibrinolysis. Recent studies have suggested that increased level of it in plasma (> 30 mg/dl) has been found to be associated with increased risk of coronary heart diseases.

Q.110. What is the effect of 'Yoga' on atherosclerosis?

Ans. 'Yoga' may help prevent coronary artery disease and stop it or even reverse the progression of atherosclerosis.

Q.111. What are the risk factors and defining levels of various biochemical values and other parameters of coronary heart disease (CHD)?

Ans.

Risk Factor	Defining Level
Abdominal obesity	Waist circumference
Men	>102 cm (> 40 inches)
Women	> 88 cm (> 35 inches)
Triglycerides	≥ 150 mg/dl
HDL cholesterol	
Men	< 40 mg/dl
Women	< 50 mg/dl
Blood pressure	> 130/> 85 mmHg
Fasting glucose	> 110 mg/dl

Q.112. How would you manage 'overweight' and 'obesity' of an individual suffering from CHD and hypercholesterolaemia?

Ans. **Weight control** – Overweight and obesity are recognized as major underlying risk factors for CHD and identified as direct targets of intervention.

Regular physical activity reduces very low density lipoprotein (VLDL) levels, raises HDL cholesterol, and in some persons, lowers LDL levels. It also can lower blood pressure, reduce insulin resistance, and favourably influence cardiovascular function. Therefore, regular physical activity becomes a routine component in the management of high serum cholesterol.

Q.113. What is phrynoderma?

Ans. Phrynoderma (**toadskin**) is an essential fatty acid disorder which is characterized by the presence of horny eruptions on the posterior and the lateral parts of the limbs, on the back and the buttocks.

Q.114. What is saponification?

Ans. The hydrolysis of triacylglycerols by alkali to produce glycerol and soaps is known as saponification.

Q.115. What is the importance of dipalmityl lecithin?

Ans. It prevents the adherence of inner surface of lungs due to surface tension. Absence of this phospholipid results in respiratory distress syndrome in infants.

Q.116. Name some important laboratory tests used for the detection of cholesterol.

Ans. (a) Salkowski test
(b) Lieberman–Burchard reaction, and
(c) Zak's test

Q.117. What are liposomes?

Ans. These have an intermittent aqueous phase in lipid bilayer and are produced when amphipathic lipids in aqueous medium are subjected to sonification. **These are now a days used extensively as carriers of drugs to target tissues.**

Q.118. What are amphipathic lipids?

Ans. The lipids which possess both hydrophobic and hydrophilic groups are known as amphipathic lipids.

Q.119. What do you understand by the term total lipids?

Ans. The term is given to the sum of the blood lipids, i.e., the sum of the:
(i) Free and ester cholesterol,
(ii) Phospholipid and
(iii) Neutral fat

Q.120. What is the normal range of total lipids in blood?

Ans. 360–820 mg%

Q.121. Which type of fat gets markedly increased in diabetes mellitus?

Ans. Neutral fat

Q.122. Name rate limiting enzymes of various cycles/pathways of lipid metabolism.

Ans.

S. No.	Cycle/pathway	Name of the enzyme
1.	Fatty acid synthesis	Acetyl CoA carboxylase (ACC)
2.	Fatty acid oxidation	Carnitine acyltransferase I (CAT 1)
3.	Ketogenesis (ketone bodies formation)	HMG-CoA synthetase
4.	Cholesterol synthesis	HMG-CoA reductase

Q.123. Who discovered the pathway 'cycle of cholesterol biosynthesis'?

Ans. Lynen

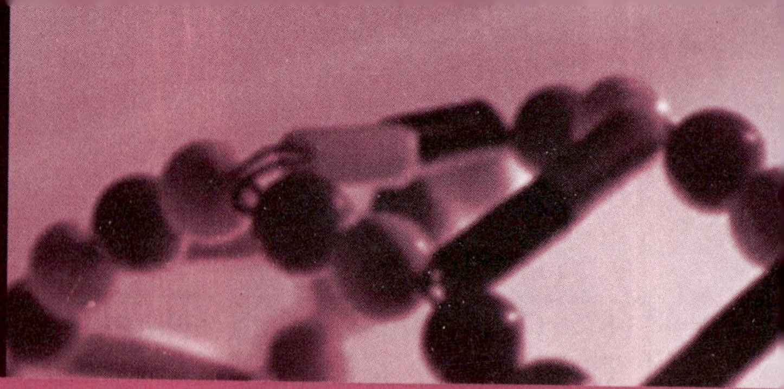

5

Proteins and their Metabolism

Q.1. Define word proteins.

Ans. Proteins have been defined as extremely complex nitrogen containing organic compounds which are found in all animal and vegetable cells, where they constitute a major part of the living protoplasm of such cells.

They are the compounds made-up of C, H, O, N and generally, sulphur and sometimes P, Fe, Cu, I, Mn, Zn and other elements.

Q.2. What are the hydrolytic products of proteins in order of decreasing complexity?

Ans. Proteoses, Peptones, Polypeptides and Amino acids.

Q.3. What are amino acids?

Ans. They are composed of an amino group ($-NH_2$), a carboxyl group ($-COOH$), a hydrogen atom, and a distinctive side chain, all bonded to a carbon atom (the α–carbon atom).

$$\begin{array}{c} NH_2 \\ \alpha\ | \\ R-C-COOH \\ | \\ H \end{array}$$

α-amino acid

Q.4. What are glycogenic (glucogenic) amino acids?

Ans. Those amino acids which give rise to the intermediates of carbohydrate metabolism are called as the glycogenic amino acids.

Q.5. Name glycogenic (glucogenic) amino acids.

Ans. Alanine, arginine, aspartic acid, glycine, histidine, proline, cysteine, glutamic acid, serine, leucine, threonine, methionine, etc.

Q.6. What are ketogenic amino acids?

Ans. Ketogenic amino acids are those which give rise to acetyl CoA during its course of metabolism.

Q.7. Name any ketogenic amino acid.

Ans. Leucine

Q.8. Name some amino acids which are both glycogenic and ketogenic.

Ans. (i) Phenylalanine
(ii) Tryptophan
(iii) Tyrosine
(iv) Isoleucine, and
(v) Lysine

Q.9. Give the classification of amino acids.

Ans. (i) Neutral amino acids :
- (a) Aliphatic amino acids : Glycine, alanine, serine, isoleucine, threonine, valine and leucine
- (b) Aromatic amino acids : Phenylalanine and tyrosine
- (c) Sulphur containing amino acids : Cysteine, cystine and methionine
- (d) Heterocyclic amino acids : Tryptophan, proline and hydroxyproline

(ii) Acidic amino acids : Aspartic acid and glutamic acid
(iii) Basic amino acids : Histidine, lysine, hydroxylysine and arginine.

Q.10. Name any three glycoproteins.

Ans. (i) Ovomucoid,
(ii) Seromucoid,
(iii) Seroglycoid, etc.

Q.11. Which method is generally used for the determination of amino acids?

Ans. Ion-exchange chromatography

Q.12. Who determined the amino acids sequence of protein bovine insulin and in which year?

Ans. Chemist Frederick Sanger (Great Britain) in the year 1958.

Q.13. What does the deficiency of essential amino acids cause?

Ans. It leads to negative nitrogen balance.

Q.14. What are the sources of amino acids in the blood?

Ans. (i) Tissue protein breakdown,
(ii) Dietary proteins,
(iii) Intracellular synthesis.

Q.15. What is the role of amino acids?

Ans. (i) As building blocks of proteins
(ii) As precursors of:
- (a) Hormones
- (b) Porphyrins
- (c) Purines
- (d) Pyrimidines
- (e) Certain vitamins like folic acid, pantothenic acid, etc.

Q.16. Name the amino acid which is optically inactive.

Ans. Glycine

Q.17. What is active methionine?

Ans. S-adenosyl methionine (SAM)

Q.18. What is the role of methionine?

Ans. As methyl group donor.

Q.19. Which amino acid gives rise to nicotinic acid during its metabolism?

Ans. Tryptophan.

Q.20. What are proteins?

Ans. Proteins are polypeptides, formed by the linking of amino acids through peptide bonds.

Q.21. Name some short chain peptides which are hormones.

Ans. (i) Vasopressin
(ii) Oxytocin

Q.22. Name any long chain peptide which is a hormone.

Ans. ACTH

Q.23. Name some such proteins which possess helical structure.

Ans. (i) Hemoglobin
(ii) Myoglobin

Q.24. Give the classification of proteins.

Ans. (i) Simple proteins
(a) Fibrous (insoluble) proteins : examples are collagens, elastins and keratins.
(b) Globular (soluble) proteins: examples are albumins and globulins
(c) Denatured proteins
(ii) Conjugated proteins
(a) Nucleoproteins
(b) Mucoproteins and glycoproteins
(c) Phosphoproteins
(d) Chromoproteins
(e) Metalloproteins
(f) Lipoproteins

Q.25. What is the configuration of amino acids present in the naturally occurring proteins?

Ans. L-configuration

Q.26. What is Biuret?

Ans. It's a compound formed by heating of two molecules of urea.

Q.27. What are the general tests for proteins?

Ans. (i) Biuret test
(ii) Ninhydrin test

Q.28. Which group is specific for Biuret reaction?

Ans. Peptide group

Q.29. What is the criteria for Biuret reaction?

Ans. Minimum two peptide groups should be present to give the test positive.

Q.30. What are the various levels of protein structure?

Ans. (i) Primary structure
(ii) Secondary structure
(iii) Tertiary structure
(iv) Quaternary structure

Q.31. What does the primary structure of protein indicate?

Ans. It refers to the sequence of individual amino acids in the polypeptide chain or chains that comprise the proteins and the location of disulphide bonds if they are present.

Q.32. What is an α-helix?

Ans. The coiling of polypeptide chain into a right handed helix.

Q.33. What is electrophoresis?

Ans. Migration of charged molecules under the influence of electricity is called electrophoresis.

Q.34. What is isoelectric point (pI) of a protein?

Ans. It is that pH at which it does not migrate either to cathode or anode. The net charge on the molecule is zero.

Q.35. Why proteins are amphoteric in nature?

Ans. Proteins contain some free amino and carboxyl groups as a result of which they give the tests for both i.e. acid and basic groups, hence they are amphoteric in nature.

Q.36. What is denaturation of proteins?

Ans. This is defined as the loss in secondary, tertiary and quaternary (if present) structures of proteins on heating. It results in loss of biological activity of the proteins.

Q.37. What is renaturation of proteins?

Ans. In this process denatured proteins may, under certain conditions be restored to proteins with many of the properties of the original protein.

Q.38. What is nitrogen balance?

Ans. If the ratio of N (i.e. protein) intake to N eliminated is equal to 1, the person is said to be in a nitrogen balance.

$$\frac{\text{N intake}}{\text{N eliminated}} = 1$$

Q.39. What is transamination?

Ans This process is referred to, in which there is transfer of an amino group of an amino acid to a keto acid as a result of which the latter changes into a new amino acid whereas the original amino acid becomes a new keto acid as shown below :

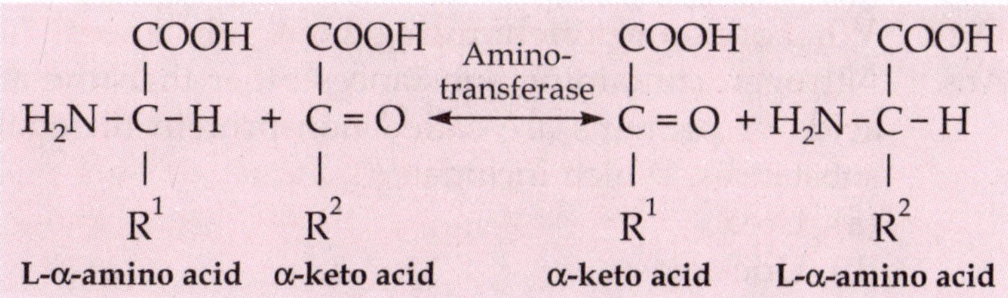

Q.40. What is deamination?

Ans. Removal of an amino group of amino acids is referred to as deamination.

Q.41. What is oxidative deamination?

Ans. In this process, there is direct removal of the amino group of the amino acids as ammonia. Besides this, there is also simultaneous oxidation of the amino acid to a keto acid, hence the name given as oxidative deamination.

Q.42. Which cofactor is required for transamination reactions?

Ans. Pyridoxal phosphate

Q.43. Name the amino acids which participate most in transamination reactions.

Ans. (i) Alanine
(ii) Aspartic acid
(iii) Glutamic acid

Q.44. How albumin and globulin are separated from each other?

Ans. Albumin can be separated by full saturation of ammonium sulphate, whereas, globulin can be separated by half saturation of ammonium sulphate.

Q.45. Name some biologically active peptides.

Ans. (i) Oxytocin
(ii) Vasopressin
(iii) Glutathione
(iv) Gramicidin-S

Q.46. Which amino acid gives rise to thyroxine?

Ans. Tyrosine

Q.47. What is the fate of ammonia?

Ans. (i) Synthesis of urea (urea cycle)
(ii) Glutamine synthesis

Q.48. What are non-protein nitrogenous substances?

Ans. Nitrogen containing substances other than the amino acids or proteins are called non-protein nitrogenous substances. Which include:

(a) Urea
(b) Uric acid
(c) Creatine
(d) Purine
(e) Pyrimidine
(f) Ammonia, etc.

Q.49. Name the amino acids involved in the synthesis of creatine.

Ans. (i) Glycine
(ii) Arginine
(iii) Methionine (as S-adenosyl methionine)

Q.50. What is the role of creatine phosphate?

Ans. As a source of energy in the contraction of muscles.

Q.51. What are the uses (roles) of glycine?

Ans. It is involved in the synthesis of:

(i) Haem
(ii) Creatine
(iii) Purines
(iv) Bile acids
(v) Proteins
(vi) Glutathione
(vii) Serine

Q.52. What is the major non-protein nitrogenous constituent of the urine?

Ans. Urea

Q.53. What is the first step of urea cycle?

Ans. The first step in the urea cycle is the formation of carbamoyl phosphate which is formed by the condensation of 1 molecule each of ammonium ion, CO_2 and phosphate (derived from ATP), reaction is catalysed by carbamoyl phosphate synthetase in the presence of magnesium ions and *N*-acetyl glutamate as a cofactor.

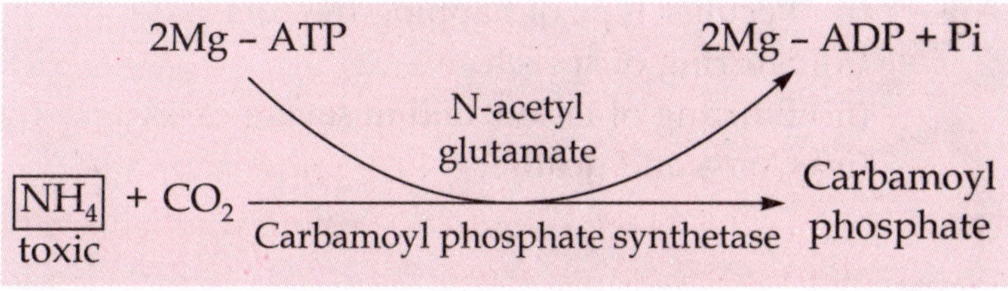

Q.54. What is the full form of GABA? How is this formed? What is the coenzyme of this reaction?

Ans. (i) GABA is γ-amino butyric acid, important in the metabolism of brain.
(ii) It is formed by the decarboxylation of glutamic acid.
(iii) Coenzyme of the reaction is pyridoxal phosphate.

Q.55. Is urea a toxic substance?

Ans. No

Q.56. Is ammonia a toxic substance?

Ans. Yes

Q.57. What are other names of urea cycle?

Ans. (i) Ornithine cycle (ii) Kreb's Henseleit cycle.

Q.58. What is the main site of urea formation?

Ans. Liver

Q.59. How is urea synthesized in the human body?

Ans. Starting substances are CO_2 and NH_3 from which carbamoyl phosphate $\longrightarrow$ Citrulline $\longrightarrow$Arginine $\longrightarrow$Urea

Q.60. Besides liver being the main site of urea formation, what are the other minor sites?

Ans. Kidney and brain

Q.61. What is the major fate of ammonia and amino groups removed from amino acids?

Ans. Formation of urea is the major fate.

Q.62. How is ammonia stored in the kidney?

Ans. In the form of glutamine which is synthesized in the kidneys from glutamic acid with the help of enzyme glutamine synthetase.

Q.63. What are the effects of ammonia intoxication?

Ans. (i) Peculiar type of flapping tremors
(ii) Slurring of speech
(iii) Blurring of vision, and in severe cases
(iv) Coma and death.

Q.64. Name the special products formed by the metabolism of aromatic amino acids.

Ans.

(i) Phenylalanine → Tyrosine → Melanin pigment, Epinephrine, Norepinephrine, Thyroxine

(ii) Tryptophan → Nicotinamide, Serotonin, Indoles

Q.65. What are the metabolic disorders of the urea cycle?

Ans. (i) Hyperammonemia type I
(ii) Hyperammonemia type II
(iii) Citrullinemia
(iv) Argininosuccinicaciduria
(v) Hyperargininemia.

Q.66. What is Phenylketonuria?

Ans. Deficiency/absence of enzyme **phenylalanine hydroxylase** in the metabolism of phenylalanine leads to **phenylketonuria** which causes *mental retardation.* One finds appreciable amount of phenylketone body (phenylpyruvic acid) in the urine of such individuals.

Q.67. What is Tyrosinosis?

Ans. Deficiency/absence of enzyme ***p*-hydroxy-phenylpyruvate oxidase** in the metabolism of tyrosine leads to *tyrosinosis.*

Q.68. What is Alkaptonuria?

Ans. Deficiency/absence of enzyme **homogentisic oxidase** in the metabolism of tyrosine leads to **alkaptonuria.** Homogentisic acid excreted in the urine may turn black upon standing.

Q.69. What is Albinism?

Ans. Deficiency/absence of enzyme **tyrosinase** in the metabolism of tyrosine leads to **albinism** in which natural melanin pigment of hair, skin and eyes is not formed.

Q.70. Name some biological important amines.

Ans. (i) Histamine
(ii) GABA
(iii) Epinephrine (adrenaline)
(iv) Norepinephrine (noradrenaline).

Q.71. What are catecholamines?

Ans. (i) Adrenaline
(ii) Noradrenaline
(iii) Dopamine.

Q.72. In phenylketonuria, besides phenylketone body, what are the other abnormal metabolites which are excreted in the urine?

Ans. (i) Phenyllactic acid (ii) Phenylacetic acid

Q.73. How will you detect the presence of phenylketonuria?

Ans. The diagnostic test is based upon the typical green colour resulting from the reaction between ferric chloride and phenylpyruvic acid.

Q.74. What do you know about homocystinuria?

Ans. (i) It is probably the second most common inborn error of amino acid metabolism, following phenylketonuria in incidence.

(ii) It is invariably associated with the dislocation of the lens of the eye (**ectopia lentis**), skeletal changes (**osteoporosis**) and cardiovascular disease (**thromboembolism**).

Q.75. What is Maple syrup urine disease?

Ans. (i) The most striking feature of this hereditary disease is the characteristic odour of the urine, which resembles that of maple syrup or burnt sugar.

(ii) Disease is characterized by very high levels of branched chain amino acids i.e. leucine, isoleucine and valine and their corresponding α-keto acids in the plasma and urine.

(iii) This is caused due to the absence or deficiency of the enzyme α-keto acid decarboxylase which catalyzes conversion of all the three branched chain α-keto acids.

Q.76. What is the site of protein synthesis?

Ans. Ribosomes

Q.77. What is the process of protein synthesis?

Ans. It involves three stages, namely :

(i) Initiation (ii) Elongation

(iii) Termination

Q.78. Name the antibiotics that inhibit protein synthesis.

Ans. (i) Chloramphenicol

(ii) Streptomycin

(iii) Tetracycline

(iv) Puromycin

(v) Cycloheximide, etc.

Q.79. What is the principal source of ammonia?

Ans. Principal source of NH_3 is the oxidation of glutamate by glutamate dehydrogenase

$$\text{Glutamic acid} \xrightarrow[\text{dehydrogenase}]{\text{Glutamate}} \alpha\text{-ketoglutaric acid} + NH_3$$

$$NAD^+ \rightarrow NADH + H^+$$

Q.80. What are the other end products of protein metabolism besides the major end product i.e. urea?

Ans. (i) Ammonia,

(ii) Creatinine, and

(iii) Uric acid

Q.81. What does HPLC mean?

Ans. High performance liquid chromatography.

Q.82. Name some amino acids with aliphatic nonpolar side chains.

Ans. Glycine, alanine, valine, leucine, and isoleucine.

Q.83. Name some amino acids with aromatic side chains.

Ans. Phenylalanine, tyrosine and tryptophan.

Q.84. Name some amino acids with hydroxyl containing side chains.

Ans. Serine and threonine.

Q.85. Name some amino acids with acidic side chains.

Ans. Aspartate and glutamate.

Q.86. Name some non-essential amino acids.

Ans. Asparagine and glutamine.

Q.87. Name some amino acids with basic side chains.

Ans. Lysine, arginine and histidine.

Q.88. Name some amino acids with sulphur containing side chains.

Ans. Cysteine, cystine, methionine and homocysteine.

Q.89. Name any imino acid.

Ans. Proline

Q.90. Name abnormalities of collagen synthesis.

Ans. Following diseases can occur as a result of defective synthesis of collagen.

Sl. No.	Disease	Effects (Symptoms)	Cause
1.	**Osteogenesis imperfecta** (brittle bone syndrome). It is further of different types: **Type I** Osteogenesis imperfecta tarda **Type- II** Osteogenesis imperfecta congenita	Causes extremely fragile bones, thin skin and weak tendons. In such cases, bones bend easily & get fractured easily. It takes place in early infancy with fractures secondary to minor trauma This type is more serious & patients generally die in utero or in the neonatal period of pulmonary hypoplasia	Mutation in the gene for either the pro-1 or pro-2-α-chains of type I collagen (Each caused by a different genetic defect)

2.	**Ehlers-Danlos syndrome** (It's a group of connective tissue disorders of which there are at least 10 types known. Most of them are genetic disorders, of which there is currently no treatment, however, in type VI, some patients have a mutant form of **lysyl hydroxylase** which respond well to vitamin C therapy)	This is caused due to inheritable defects in the metabolism of fibrillar collagen molecules. Such patients have **hyperflexible joints** and **highly** extensible skin & exhibit defects in collagen type I & type III fibrils.	Deficiency/ missing of enzyme **lysyl hydroxy-lase or procollagen peptidase**
3.	**Alport syndrome**	In this disease, glomerular basement membrane gets disrupted (it is an inherited kidney disease)	Mutation in type IV collagen gene

Q.91. What is actin?

Ans. Actin is a polymer of globular–shaped subunits (called G-actin), which are 43,000 MW in size. One molecule of ATP is bound to each G-actin.

Q.92. What are the functions of actin protein?

Ans. Actin and its isoforms are involved in different cellular movement processes and contractile functions.

Q.93. What is troponin?

Ans. It is a 73,000 MW complex of three polypeptides : troponin-T, troponin-I and troponin-C. There is one troponin complex for every tropomyosin.

Q.94. Which compound acts as a means of trapping and transporting free ammonia which is very toxic?

Ans. Glutamine.

Q.95. What are the functions of troponin?

Ans. The troponin complex in conjunction with tropomyosin mediates the regulation of contraction by calcium. Each polypeptide of the troponin complex exhibits a different activity that is essential to the over all function of the complex:

(a) Troponin-T binds to tropomyosin
(b) Troponin-I binds to actin
(c) Troponin-C binds to calcium.

Q.95A. How is melanin formed in the melanocytes?

Ans. It is formed by the action of enzyme tyrosinase on tyrosine:

$$\text{Tyrosine} \xrightarrow{\text{Tyrosinase}} \text{Melanin}$$

When the enzyme is not present, the skin has no pigment (albinism).

Q.96. What is the diagnostic application of homocysteine?

Ans. While high levels of homocysteine (hyperhomocysteinemia) have been found to be associated with cardiovascular, renal diseases, etc., there are reports of its low levels (hypohomocysteinemia) in pregnancy.

Q.97. How δ-aminolevulinic acid (ALA) is synthesized and what is its importance?

Ans. Glycine and succinyl CoA condense to form ALA which is responsible for the synthesis of haem.

Q.98. What are chaperone?

Ans. Molecular chaperone represent a diverse class of protein molecules. These chaperones function by inhibiting incorrect interactions, which are often possible in their absence. Some molecular chaperones (but not all of them) are also **stress proteins,** so that it is possible that all **stress proteins act as molecular chaperones.**

Q.99. By what term active sulfate is known as?

Ans. PAPS (Phosphoadenosine phospho-5-sulphate)

Q.100. How PAPS is formed?

Ans. It's formed by the reaction between ATP and SO_4 when the sulfate is attached to the ribose -5′ phosphate.

$$ATP + SO_4^- \longrightarrow PAPS + PPi$$

Q.101. In which type of reactions, PAPS is used?

Ans. PAPS is used for various sulfuration reactions, e.g.

(i) Synthesis of sulfatides,

(ii) Synthesis of GAG, (glycosaminoglycans) etc.

Q.102. How many forms of presentation of cystinosis are there?

Ans. There are three forms of presentation, namely;

(a) Infantile, where renal failure is seen in the first decade.

(b) Juvenile, in which renal failure appears in the second decade, and

(c) Adult benign type where kidneys are spared, and deposition of cystine are mainly seen in cornea. There is found an abnormality in the transport of cystine which is responsible for the accumulation.

Q.103. What are the clinical manifestations of cystinosis?

Ans. Clinical manifestations include renal symptoms, vitamin-D resistant rickets, acidosis, polyuria, dehydration and **renal failure.** Corneal deposits may lead to photophobia, itching and headache. **It is a rare familial storage disorder which is characterized by the deposition of cystine crystals in various body tissues, like liver, spleen, kidneys, bone marrow, cornea, etc.**

Q.104. What is the treatment of cystinosis?

Ans. Treatment consists in giving such patients adequate fluid so as to increase urinary output, correction of acidosis by sodium bicarbonate, supplementation of vitamin-D and calcium to combat rickets as well as administration of **thiol reagents such as D-penicillamine.**

Q.105. What are the causes of hypermethioninemia?

Ans. Causes are :

a) Protein rich diet,
b) Impaired utilization,
c) Excessive remethylation of homocysteine, and
d) Secondary to hepatic dysfunction

Biochemical abnormality is the **block in the utilization of homocysteine to methionine.**

Q.106. What is Oasthouse syndrome?

Ans. **This syndrome is due to malabsorption of methionine. The children excrete in urine the following:**

a) Methionine,
b) Aromatic amino acids, and
c) Branched chain keto acids

Q.107. What is the importance of serum electrophoresis pattern of proteins?

Ans. It is used for the diagnosis of certain diseases:

(i) In multiple myeloma : A sharp and **distinct M-band appears in the γ-globulin** fraction
(ii) In nephrotic syndrome : Albumin is decreased with a prominent α_2–globulin fraction.
(iii) In primary immune deficiency: **γ–Globulin band is diminished.**

Q.108. What is A/G ratio and what is its significance?

Ans. A/G ratio expresses their relation in serum concentration and its normal range is 1.2 to 1.5.

(i) A/G ratio gets lowered (due to decrease in albumin) in liver diseases.
(ii) A/G ratio gets increased (due to increase in globulins) in chronic infections.

Q.109. What is the diagnostic importance of α_1–antitrypsin?

Ans. α_1-antitrypsin (α_1-antiproteinase) is a component of γ-globulins. Its deficiency has been found to be associated in emphysema (**abnormal distension of lungs**).

Q.110. What do you know about haptoglobin?

Ans. Haptoglobin (Hp) is a plasma glycoprotein. It binds with the free hemoglobin that spills into the plasma due to hemolysis.

Q.111. What is ceruloplasmin and its importance?

Ans. It is a blue coloured, copper containing α_2–globulin. It gets decreased in **Wilson'disease** and its normal plasma level is around 30 mg/dl.

Q.112. What do you understand by immunity?

Ans. The higher organisms including humans have evolved a defense system collectively referred to as immunity, in order to protect themselves against the invasion of foreign substances i.e., microorganisms, viruses or proteins. Two types of immunity have been identified:

(a) **Cellular Immunity :** It is mediated by T-lymphocytes (T-cells) that defends the body against the invasion of parasites, fungi, foreign tissues, etc.

(b) **Humoral Immunity :** It is mediated by a special group of proteins known as immunoglobulins or antibodies. The β-lymphocytes or β-cells are responsible for the production of immunoglobulins.

Q.113. What are immunoglobulins?

Ans. These are a specialized group of glycoproteins synthesized by β-cells. The basic structure of an immunoglobulin consists of two identical heavy (H) chains and two identical light (L) chains held together by disulfide linkages. Each chain (H or L) of Ig has constant and variable regions. Human beings have 5 classes of Ig, i.e., IgG, IgA, IgM, IgD and IgE, each one with a distinct heavy chain (respectively G, A, M, D, E) and a specific function. Functions of different immunoglobulins are :

(i) IgG is involved in the destruction of foreign cells.

(ii) IgA prevents the foreign substance from entering the body.

(iii) IgM is most effective against invading micro-organisms

(iv) IgD is β-cell receptor

(v) IgE is involved in allergic reactions.

Q.114. What is multiple myeloma?

Ans. Multiple myeloma, a plasma cell cancer, constitutes nearly 1% of all cancers affecting population. This decrease is characterized by the abnormal production of immunoglobulins (mostly IgG). On electrophoresis of plasma proteins, a distinct M-bond is observed in the patients of multiple myeloma.

Q.115. What are Bence Jones proteins and how are they detected?

Ans. These are the light (κ an λ) chains immunoglobulins which are synthesized in plenty. In about 20% of multiple myeloma patients, these are excreted in urine.

Bence Jones proteins can be detected either by electrophoresis or heat test.

Bence Jones protein may be distinguished from other proteins found in urine as it will precipitate between 40-60°C, whereas other proteins precipitate between 60-70°C. On raising the temperature higher than 60°C, Bence Jones protein redissolves, but other proteins do not. On cooling to 60°C from boiling, it reprecipitates. It is a non-blood protein and is believed to be of diagnostic importance in cases of :

(a) multiple myeloma, and

(b) myelogenic osteosarcoma.

Q.116. What do you know about anticoagulants?

Ans. These are the substances that check the clotting of blood. These include oxalate, heparin, EDTA and citrate, which can bind with Ca^{++} and are very effective as anticoagulants. Heparin is a natural anticoagulant (secreted by mast cells) that maintains normal blood homeostasis.

Q.117. What are the major abnormalities associated with blood clotting?

Ans. Defects in clotting factors are responsible for abnormalities in blood clotting, for e.g.,

(i) Hemophilia-A (defect - **antihemophilic factor i.e., VII**)

(ii) Hemophilia-B or Christmas disease (defect-**Christmas factor, i.e., IX**)

Q.118. How are the amino acids classified from the metabolic point of view?

Ans. Based on metabolic fate, these have been divided into three categories:

a) **Glycogenic :** Those amino acids which act as precursors for the synthesis of glucose (or glycogen), e.g., alanine aspartate, glycine.

b) **Ketogenic :** Those amino acids which have got the capability to synthesize fat, e.g., leucine, lysine.

c) **Glycogenic and Ketogenic, both :** Those amino acids which have got the capability to synthesize both glucose and fats, e.g., isoleucine, phenylalanine and lysine.

Q.119. What do you understand by non-protein amino acids?

Ans. These are the amino acids which are never found in protein structure and are collectively referred to as non-protein amino acids, e.g., **ornithine, citrulline, thyroxine,** etc. They perform several very important biological functions in the body.

Q.120. Name some non-α-amino acids.

Ans. (a) β - Alanine

(b) γ - Aminobutyric acid

(c) δ - Aminolevulinic acid

(d) β - Aminoisobutyric acid

Q.121. What is Sanger's reagent & its importance?

Ans. It is chemically 1-fluoro–2, 4-dinitrobenzene (FDNB) which is used to detect the N-terminal amino acid of a polypeptide or a protein.

Q.122. What do you understand by salting out?

Ans. It is the process of the precipitation of protein by the addition of neutral salts such as ammonium sulfate or sodium sulfate.

Q.123. What is the importance of salting out?

Ans. The importance of this process/technique is for the separation of several proteins in the laboratory, e.g., serum albumins and serum globulins.

Q.124 What is salting in?

Ans. In this process, there is addition of small quantities of neutral salts which increases the solubility of proteins.

Q.125. What are the important functions of glutathione?

Ans. It is a tripeptide (Glu-Cys-Gly) which plays very important functions in the body, namely:

(i) It maintains the sulfhydryl groups (-SH) in proteins.
(ii) It is involved in the transport of certain amino acids in the intestine and kidney.
(iii) It maintains the structure and integrity of the erythrocyte membrane.
(iv) It protects hemoglobin from getting oxidized.

Q.126. What are glycoproteins?

Ans. The proteins structurally associated with the carbohydrates are referred to as glycoproteins (conjugated protein i.e., conjugation of protein with carbohydrate)

Q.127. What are antifreeze glycoproteins?

Ans. Those glycoproteins which have a tendency to lower the freezing point of water and interfere with the crystal formation of ice. The **'Antarctic fishes' living below –200°C contain antifreeze glycoproteins which are responsible for their survival.**

Q.128. What is the chemical name of creatine?

Ans. Methylguanido acetic acid.

Q.129 What is creatinine?

Ans. It is an anhydride of creatine.

Q.130 In which form, creatine is found in muscles?

Ans. Creatine phosphate (found in muscles only and not in any other tissue).

Q.131. What is the other name for creatine phosphate?

Ans. Phosphagen

Q.132. What is the approximate percentage of creatine in muscles?

Ans. 0.5%

Q.133. From which amino acids creatine is formed in animal tissues?

Ans. (a) Glycine
(b) Arginine and
(c) Methionine

Q.134. Name such muscles diseases in which creatinuria is found.

Ans. (a) Poliomyelitis

(b) Muscular dystrophies, etc.

Q.135. What do you understand by proteoglycans?

Ans. They are the complexes formed of proteins and glycosaminoglycans.

Q.136. Name the rate limiting enzyme of urea cycle.

Ans. Carbamoyl phosphate synthetase-I

Q.137. Name the affected proteins in case of sufferers of cataract.

Ans. Crystallins.

Q.138. What do you mean by the term 'standard amino acids'.

Ans. Generally, a protein is made-up of 20 regular amino acids which are responsible for the biosynthesis of protein (these infact get incorporated into a protein). This is because only these 20 amino acids possess **genetic code** which specify the composition and size of a protein. Therefore, these are called standard amino acids.

Q.139. What is genetic code?

Ans. It is the three nucleotide base sequence which codes for amino acids and determines the sequence of amino acids in proteins. The genetic code is **universal** in nature (i.e., a particular amino acid is coded by the same codon in proteins of all organisms).

Q.140. What are polar (hydrophilic) amino acids?

Ans. Amino acids with ionizable groups (amino acids possessing charged groups) are polar.

Q.141. What are hydrophilic amino acids?

Ans. Acidic amino acids like aspartate, glutamate (with negatively charged groups) and basic amino acids like lysine, arginine and histidine (with positively charged groups) are strongly hydrophilic (water loving).

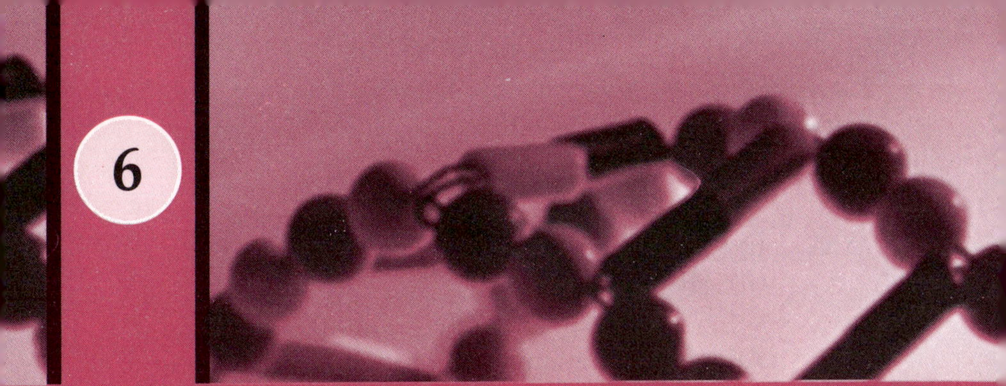

6

Nucleic Acids and Their Metabolism

Q.1. Name some eminent personalities who have contributed a lot in the field of nucleic acids.

Ans. (i) Watson,

(ii) Crick,

(iii) Hargobind Khorana,

(iv) Chargaff, and

(v) Davidson, etc.

Q.2. Name any India-born scientist who has worked a lot on nucleic acids.

Ans. Dr. Hargobind Khorana.

Q.3. For what contribution Dr. Hargobind Khorana was awarded Nobel Prize and in which year?

Ans. He succeeded in synthesizing the first wholly artificial gene. He also interpreted genetic code and its function in the protein synthesis for which he was awarded Nobel Prize in 1968.

Q.4. How many types of nucleic acids are there?

Ans. (i) Deoxyribonucleic acid (DNA), and

(ii) Ribonucleic acid (RNA).

Q.5. What are the sugars of DNA and RNA?

Ans. D-deoxyribose and d-ribose respectively.

Q.6. Name the proteins of nucleoproteins.

Ans. (i) Protamines, and
(ii) Histones.

Q.7. What are the major purine nucleotides of DNA?

Ans. Adenine and guanine.

Q.8. What are nucleic acids?

Ans. (i) They are polymers of nucleotides.
(ii) They are made-up of nitrogenous bases, sugars and phosphoric acid.
(iii) These are macromolecules which are strongly acidic in nature at physiological pH.

Q.9. What are the main functions of nucleic acids?

Ans. (1) They transmit hereditary characters from one offspring to another.
(ii) They direct the synthesis of proteins.
(iii) They control the synthesis of enzymes.
(iv) They are involved in the causation of cancer (malignancy).

Q.10. How many types of nitrogenous bases are there?

Ans. Two types, either :
(i) Purine or
(ii) Pyrimidine.

Q.11. Name the principal purine bases found in the nucleic acids.

Ans. (i) Adenine, and
(ii) Guanine.

Q.12. Name the principal pyrimidine bases of nucleic acids.

Ans. (i) Thymine, and
(ii) Cytosine.

Q.13. Where does DNA remain present in the cell?

Ans. (i) It remains present in chromosomes and constitutes genes.
(ii) Mitochondria do also possess some DNA.

Q.14. Of how many deoxyribonucleotides a DNA molecule is formed of?

Ans. Each DNA molecule is a polymer of 20,000 or more deoxyribonucleotides.

Q.15. What is the molecular weight of DNA?

Ans. 1.6×10^6 to 2×10^9

Q.16. By which bond nucleotides remain connected to each other?

Ans. Phosphate diester bond.

Q.17. What are the major pyrimidine nucleotides of DNA?

Ans. Thymine and cytosine.

Q.18. What is a nucleoside?

Ans. A combination of sugar and nitrogenous base is called a nucleoside.

Q.19. Who discovered the double helical structure of DNA molecule?

Ans. Watson and Crick that is why it's also popularly known as Watson Crick model.

Q.20. In which year Watson and Crick were awarded Nobel Prize for their brilliant discovery of double helical structure of DNA molecule?

Ans. 1962.

Q.21. What is the base-pairing rule?

Ans. (i) Adenine will combine with thymine.
(ii) Guanine will combine with cytosine.

Q.22. What is the number of hydrogen bonds present between (i) Adenine and Thymine, (ii) Guanine and Cytosine?

Ans. (i) Two hydrogen bonds
(ii) Three hydrogen bonds.

Q.23. How the two coiled strands of the double-helix remain held together?

Ans. By hydrogen bonds.

Q.24. What is DNA?

Ans. DNA may be regarded as the master tape of the cell, the computer programme in which all the information required for the operation of the cell and its reproduction remains contained.

Q.25. What do you know about the structure of a DNA molecule?

Ans. (i) It has got double stranded helical structure.
(ii) It is formed by the twisting of two linear polydeoxyribonucleotide strands in opposite directions and around one another.
(iii) Both the strands of the helix form right handed coils but they are antiparallel to one another.

Q.26. What is a nucleotide?

Ans. A combination of sugar-nitrogenous base and phosphate is called a nucleotide.

Q.27. What is the difference between DNA and RNA?

Ans.

	DNA	RNA
(i)	**Bases** present are adenine, guanine, cytosine and thymine	**Bases** present are adenine, guanine, cytosine and uracil
(ii)	**Sugar** present is deoxyribose	**Sugar** present is ribose
(iii)	It's a double strand molecule	It's a single strand molecule

Q.28. What are the various types of RNA?

Ans. RNA has three types, i.e.
(i) Messenger RNA (m-RNA)
(ii) Transfer RNA (t-RNA) or soluble RNA (s-RNA), and
(iii) Ribosomal RNA (r-RNA).

Q.29. Where RNA remains located in the cell?

Ans. It remains located in the:
(i) Nucleolus,
(ii) Ribosomes, and
(iii) Mitochondria.

Q.30. Of how many ribonucleotides, a RNA molecule is formed of?

Ans. Less than 75 to more than 3,500.

Q.31. How ribonucleotides remain connected to each other?

Ans. By phosphate diester bonds.

Q.32. What is the function of m-RNA?

Ans. They carry message from nuclear DNA to ribosomes (site

of protein synthesis) as to when they should synthesize various important substances like enzymes, proteins, polypeptide hormones, etc.

Q.33. What is the function of transfer RNA?

Ans. Its main function is to transfer amino acid, for this purpose, it gets attached with the activated amino acid and then carries it to the site of protein synthesis so that it be added to the growing polypeptide chain.

Q.34. What is replication?

Ans. Copying of DNA to form identical daughter molecules is called the replication.

Q.35. What is transcription?

Ans. Transcription is the process by which genetic message in DNA is transcribed in the form of messenger RNA to be carried to the ribosomes.

Q.36. What is translation?

Ans. Translation is the process by which genetic message is decoded on the ribosomes.

Q.37. By which enzymes DNA is synthesized?

Ans. DNA polymerases.

Q.38. What is a triplet or codon?

Ans. It's the sequence of three non-overlapping nucleotides.

Q.39. What is genetic code?

Ans. It refers to the language used by the genetic material i.e. the DNA to transfer genetic information to the site of new product formation. Genetic code is **universal.**

Q.40. What is the chain initiating codon in protein synthesis?

Ans. AUG

Q.41. Chain initiating codon AUG codes for which amino acid in eukaryotes and prokaryotes?

Ans. (i) Methionine in eukaryotes, and
(ii) *N*-formyl methionine in prokaryotes.

Q.42. What are the chain terminating codons?

Ans. These are three, i.e.
(i) UAA
(ii) UAG, and
(iii) UGA.

Q.43. What are the sense codons?

Ans. Codons which code for an amino acid are called "sense codons".

Q.44. What are non-sense codons?

Ans. The three codons that do not code for any amino acid are called the "non-sense codons".

Q.45. By which enzyme synthesis of RNA is catalysed?

Ans. DNA-dependent RNA-polymerase.

Q.46. Does DNA direct its own synthesis?

Ans. Yes.

Q.47. Does DNA also direct the synthesis of RNA?

Ans. Yes.

Q.48. What do you understand by the term polycistronic?

Ans. More than one genetic code.

Q.49. What do you understand by the term monocistronic?

Ans. One genetic code.

Q.50. By how many codons methionine is coded? What is that code?

Ans. Only one, AUG.

Q.51. Which enzyme is found to be missing in Lesch-Nyhan syndrome?

Ans. GMP pyrophosphorylase.

Q.52. By how many codons tryptophan is coded? What is that code?

Ans. Only one, UGG.

Q.53. What is mutation?

Ans. An alteration in the sequence of purine and pyrimidine bases in a gene is called 'mutation'.

Q.54. Name some 'mutagens'.

Ans.

A	Most chemical carcinogens are mutagens, namely:	
(a)	Polycyclic aromatic hydrocarbons	3-4- Benzpyrene, methylcholanthrene, etc
(b)	Aromatic amines	2- Acetylaminofluorene
(c)	Nitrosamines	Dimethylnitrosamine

(d)	Various drugs	Alkylating agents, etc.
(e)	Naturally occurring compounds	Aflatoxins for e.g., Aflatoxin B_1, & C_1, etc.
(f)	Inorganic compounds	Arsenic, asbestos cadmium, chromium, etc.
B	Ultraviolet rays.	
C	X-rays	
D	γ-rays.	

Q.55. What are the various sources of carbon and nitrogen in purine skeleton?

Ans Aspartic acid, formate, glycine, respiratory CO_2 and amide nitrogen of glutamine.

Q.56. What is the fate of purine bases?

Ans. They are converted to uric acid.

Q.57. What is the end product of purine catabolism in humans?

Ans. Uric acid.

Q.58. What is the normal uric acid level in blood?

Ans. (i) 2.5-7.0 mg/dl (men)

(ii) 1.5-6.0 mg/dl (women).

Q.59. What is gout?

Ans. (i) Increased level of uric acid in blood gives rise to a condition known as gout.

(ii) Uric acid deposits (tophi) accumulate in the cartilages and joints and cause painful inflammatory condition in them.

Q.60. What is the drug being used in the treatment of gout?

Ans. (i) A drug **Colchicine** which interrupts the mitosis of leucocytes, and thus, prevents development of inflammation.

(ii) A competitive inhibitor of xanthine oxidase i.e. **Allopurinol** is used.

Q.61. What dietary precautions should be taken by the patients suffering from gout?

Ans. (i) They should not consume non-vegetarian dishes because they are rich in purines vis-a-vis nucleoproteins; examples of such dishes are glandular organs like liver etc.

(ii) A diet of milk, eggs and cheese (very low in purine content) causes practically no elevation in uric acid level.

Q.62. How biosynthesis of pyrimidines takes place?

Ans. It takes place from:

(i) Ammonia

(ii) CO_2 and

(iii) Aspartate.

Q.63. How are pyrimidines catabolized?

Ans. (i) Pyrimidines like cytosine and uracil are broken down to β-ureidopropionic acid and β-alanine.

(ii) Other pyrimidines like methylcytosine and thymine are converted to β-aminoisobutyric acid and succinic acid.

Q.64. Name some inhibitors of nucleic acid synthesis.

Ans. (i) Azaserine

(ii) Pteroylglutamic acid

(iii) 8-Azaguanine

(iv) Antibiotics-Anthramycin, Actinomycin-D, Mitomycin, Novobiocin, etc.

Q.65. Name one enzyme of purine metabolism which remains absent in human beings. What is its function?

Ans. Uricase which oxidizes uric acid to allantoin. This is found in lower animals, therefore, they have no hyperuricemia and gout.

Q.66. Give the schematic diagram of the catabolism of pyrimidines. (cytosine and 5-methylcytosine).

Ans.

(a)

$$\text{Cytosine} \xrightarrow{-NH_3} \text{uracil} \xrightarrow{\text{NADPH}} \text{dihydro-}$$

$$\text{uracil} \longrightarrow \beta\text{-alanine} + NH_3 + CO_2$$

(b) $\text{5-Methylcytosine} \xrightarrow{-NH_3} \text{thymine} \xrightarrow{NADPH} \text{dihydrothymine} \longrightarrow \beta\text{-aminoisobutyrate} + NH_3 + CO_2$

It may be noted that while the amino acids utilized for protein metabolism are α-amino acids but during the catabolism of pyrimidines β-amino acids are formed.

Q.67. Give schematic account of the catabolism of nucleotides i.e., adenosine and guanosine.

Ans. The catabolism of the two nucleotides i.e., adenosine and guanosine is initially different as enzyme **adenase is found to be in negligible amount in the liver, whereas guanase is found in significant amount.**

$\text{Adenosine} \xrightarrow[\text{deaminase}]{\text{Adenosine}} \text{Inosine} \xrightarrow[\text{phosphorylase}]{\text{Purine nucleoside}} \text{Hypoxanthine}$

$\text{Hypoxanthine} \xrightarrow{\text{Xanthine dehydrogenase, } O_2} \text{Xanthine}$

$\text{Guanosine} \xrightarrow[\text{phosphorylase}]{\text{Purine nucleoside}} \text{Guanine} \xrightarrow{\text{Guanase}} \text{Xanthine}$

$\text{Xanthine} \xrightarrow{\text{Xanthine dehydrogenase, } O_2} \text{Uric acid}$

Hence, uric acid is the end product of purine catabolism. When there is excessive catabolism of purine nucleosides as in cases of **leukaemia** and **polycythemia** vera, there is secondary hyperuricemia.

Q.68. What is Z-DNA (Zig zag DNA)?

Ans. This is a DNA form with a left handed double helix in which the phosphodiester backbone zigzags along the molecule; hence, the name has been given as zigzag DNA.

It is the least trusted DNA. The existence of Z-DNA in drosophilia (fruit fly) chromosomes has been established. Whereas human DNA contains potential Z-DNA left- handed helix forming regions in it, the inventor of this finding is **the Indian Biophysicist Sasisekhran.** Finding of Professor Sasisekhran is **contrary to the finding of Watson and Crick who proposed right handed DNA molecule.**

Q.69. What are point mutations?

Ans. **The classic example of point mutation is sickle cell disease**, which is caused by a mutation of a single base out of the $3x10^9$ in the genome, a T-to-A DNA substitution, which, in turn, results in an A-to-U change in the m-RNA corresponding to the sixth codon of the **β-globin** gene. The altered codon specifies a different amino acid (**valine rather** than **glutamic acid**), and this causes a structural abnormality of the β-globin gene.

Other point mutations in and around the **β-globin** gene result in decreased or in some instances, no production of **β-globin; β-thalassemia** is the result of these mutations. (The thalassemias are characterized by defects in the synthesis of hemoglobin subunits, **and so β- thalassemia results when there is an insufficient production of β-globin).**

Q.70. Name the second messengers.

Ans. (i) Cyclic AMP
(ii) Cyclic GMP
(iii) Calcium
(iv) Insulin
(v) Membrane phospholipids
(vi) Tyrosine kinase, etc.

Q.71. Name some biologically important nucleotides other than those found in nucleic acids structures.

Ans: FAD, NAD^+, $NADP^+$, Coenzyme-A, S-adenosylmethionine, UDP-glucose, etc.

Q.72. What is Chargaff's rule?

Ans. The molar equivalence between the purines and pyrimidines in DNA structure represents **Chargaff's rule i.e., A=T, G ≡ C.** The double helical structure of DNA derives its strength from Chargaff's rule.

Q.73. What are the different forms of DNA structure?

Ans. The double helical structure of DNA exists in at least 6 different forms, i.e., A, B, C, D, E and Z. Among these, A, B and Z are important. A-form has 11 base pairs per turn, B-form 10 base pairs, whereas Z-form contains 12 base pairs per turn.

Q.74. What do you understand by branched chain DNA?

Ans. Increased sensitivity can also be achieved by methods that amplify the detection or signal resulting from the hybridization assay. The branched chain DNA (b DNA) approach developed by Chiron uses a sandwich hybridization assay. Each branch has as many as three signal-generating enzymes, such as alkaline phosphatase, covalently bound.

Q.75 Name the rate limiting enzymes of various pathways of nucleic acids metabolism.

Ans.

Sl. No.	Pathway	Name of rate limiting enzyme
1.	de novo pyrimidine synthesis	Aspartate transcarbamoylase (ATCase)
2.	de novo purine synthesis	Glutamine-PRPP amidotransferase

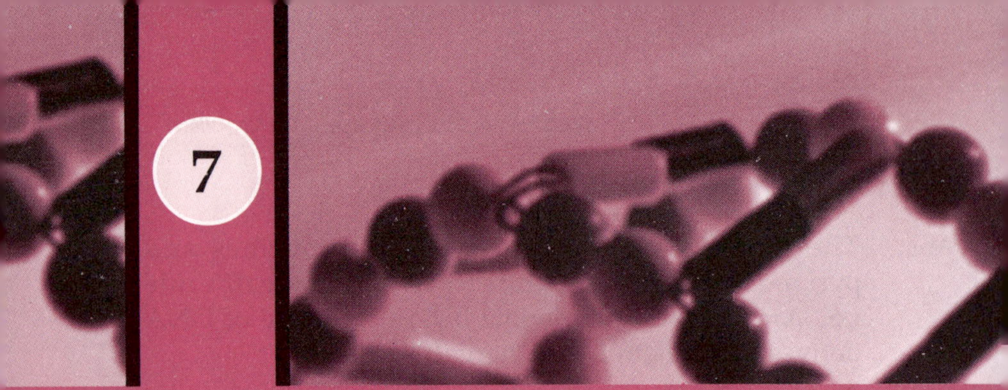

7

WATER AND MINERAL METABOLISM

Q.1. What is the percentage of water in human body?

Ans. About 65-70%.

Q.2. What is the percentage of minerals in human body?

Ans. About 8.5%.

Q.3. Name the important minerals found in the human body.

Ans. Sodium, potassium, calcium, magnesium, phosphorus, chlorine, sulphur, iron and copper, etc.

Q.4. Name the macroelements found in the body.

Ans. Ca, Mg, Na, K, P, S, Cl and Fe.

Q.5. What are the biological functions of water?

Ans.
(i) Solvent action
(ii) Ionization
(iii) Homeostasis
(iv) Fluid exchange
(v) Lubricating action
(vi) Latent heat of evaporation.

Q.6. What is the daily water (fluid) intake by drinks per day?

Ans. 2.5 - 3.5 litres

Q.7. What is the amount of metabolic water i.e., produced by oxidation of food per day?

Ans. Nearly 400 ml.

Q.8. What is the water loss by lungs per day?

Ans. Nearly 400 ml.

Q.9. What is the water loss through skin per day?

Ans. 700 ml.

Q.10. What is the water loss through urine per day?

Ans. Nearly 1250 ml.

Q.11. What is the water loss through faeces per day?

Ans. Nearly 100 ml.

Q.12. What are the daily requirements of sodium and chloride?

Ans. 5 and 7.5 g respectively.

Q.13. What is the daily requirement of potassium?

Ans. About 4 g.

Q.14. Why do we require sodium?

Ans. It helps in the following ways:

(i) Maintenance of fluid balance
(ii) Neuromuscular excitability
(iii) Active transport
(iv) Enzyme action
(v) Conduction and transmission of nerve impulses, etc.

Q.15. Why do we require potassium?

Ans. It helps in the following ways:

(i) Neuromuscular excitability
(ii) Enzyme action
(iii) Activity of cardiac muscles
(iv) Conduction and transmission of nerve impulses, etc.

Q.16. Why do we require chloride?

Ans. It helps in the following ways:

(i) Maintenance of fluid balance
(ii) Acid-base balance
(iii) Active transport
(iv) Enzyme action, etc.

Q.17. What are the sources of iron?

Ans. Liver, lentils, lettuce, spinach, radish tops, fig, egg-yolk, nuts, dates, soyabeans, etc.

Q.18. What happens after excessive loss of NaCl through sweat?

Ans. It causes:
(i) Salt cramps
(ii) Hyponatraemia with nausea
(iii) Muscle cramps, etc.

Q.19. What happens after drinking salt-free fluids?

Ans. It may cause:
(i) Hyponatremia with nausea
(ii) Muscle cramps
(iii) Diarrhoea, etc.

Q.20. Intense vomiting leads to :

Ans. (i) Chloride depletion
(ii) Fall in plasma chloride, sodium and potassium levels
(iii) Dehydration
(iv) Some of the lost Cl may be replaced by HCO_3, thus increasing the plasma bicarbonate level which may result into metabolic alkalosis.

Q.21. Why do we require magnesium?

Ans. We require it because:
(i) It's a constituent of bones and teeth.
(ii) It also plays a role in neuromuscular excitability.
(iii) It also plays a role in various enzymatic reactions as a cofactor or activator.

Q.22. Why do we require phosphorus?

Ans. We require it because:
(i) It's a constituent of bones and teeth.
(ii) It plays vital role in energy transfer.
(iii) It plays vital role in acid-base regulation.
(iv) It has got role in phosphorylation.
(v) It helps in the formation of animal products, etc.
(vi) It's also a constituent of nucleic acids.

Q.23. Why do we require calcium?

Ans. We require it because:
(1) It's a very important constituent of bones and teeth.
(ii) It's requirement gets enhanced in the infants and children as elongation of bones and the development of teeth occur in them at a faster rate.
(iii) It's also required for blood coagulation.

(iv) It acts as an enzyme activator for various biological reactions.
(v) It plays role in muscle contraction, conduction of nerve impulses, neuromuscular transmission and cardiac contraction.
(vi) It's an important constituent of milk and also helps in the secretion of milk.

Q.24 What is the daily requirement of iron for adult man, adult woman and pregnant/lactating woman?

Ans. 10, 18 and 20 mgs respectively.

Q.25. Why do we require iron?

Ans. We require it because:
(i) Its deficiency causes hypochromic microcytic anaemia, characterized by low levels of protein-bound iodine (PBI) in the plasma, low hemoglobin contents of blood and reduced cytochrome contents of tissues.
(ii) Many heme compounds participate in the transport and storage of oxygen and also in the transport of electrons during tissue oxidations. Respiratory pigments like hemoglobin and myoglobin are the important examples of such compounds.

Q.26 What is siderosis?

Ans. (i) It's an excessive accumulation of iron in the body tissues like spleen, liver, pancreas and the skin.
(ii) It's caused by the excessive intestinal absorption of iron either due to the congenital defects or habitual intake of high iron-low phosphorus diets.

Q.27. What are the symptoms of siderosis?

Ans. Symptoms include:
(i) Diabetes mellitus
(ii) Hepatic cirrhosis
(iii) Fibrosis of tissues, and
(iv) Bronzing of the skin.

Q.28. What is the daily requirement of copper?

Ans. 2.5 mg.

Q.29. What is the main storehouse of copper in the body?

Ans. Liver.

Q.30. What does iodine deficiency cause?

Ans. (i) Thyroid enlargement (iodine-deficiency goiter), the obvious sign of which is swelling in the neck.

(ii) Hypothyroidism.

Q.31. What does inborn error or hereditary defect in copper metabolism cause?

Ans. Wilson's disease (hepatolenticular degeneration).

Q.32. Why do we require copper?

Ans. We require it because:

(i) It plays a very important role in iron metabolism, i.e., it helps in the utilization of iron for the synthesis of hemoglobin.

(ii) It plays a vital role in enzymic actions.

(iii) It remains present in the prosthetic groups of the enzymes of oxidase class i.e., cytochrome oxidase, ascorbic acid oxidase, tyrosinase, MAO (mono-amine oxidase), uricase, etc.

(iv) It's also a constituent of haemocyanin.

Q.33. What is Wilson's disease?

Ans. (i) In this disease plasma ceruloplasmin level gets lowered and the uncombined Cu^{++} of plasma gets elevated.

(ii) **Copper gets deposited in damaging amounts in tissues like liver, pancreas, kidney, cornea and the lenticular nucleus of the brain which may cause abnormal muscular movements (like Parkinson's disease),** diabetes mellitus, renal tubular damage, a **visible brown ring (*Kayser-Fleischer ring*) at the margin of cornea,** hepatic cirrhosis and jaundice and the patient may ultimately die of hepatic failure.

Q.34. Is there any treatment of Wilson's disease?

Ans. Administration of D-penicillamine may cause some improvement by increasing Cu excretion.

Q.35. Name the sources of iodine.

Ans. Iodized table salt, flesh and oil of marine fishes like cod, onion and iodates added to bread etc.

Q.36. What is the daily requirement of iodine for adults?

Ans. 140 μg.

Q.37. Why do we require iodine?

Ans. It's required for the synthesis of thyroid hormones i.e. T_3 and T_4.

Q.38. What is the name of the protein in which thyroxine remains confined?

Ans. Thyroglobulin.

Q.39. What should be the ideal calcium phosphorus ratio?

Ans. 1 : 1 for ideal absorption.

Q.40. What does iodine deficiency cause?

Ans. (i) Thyroid enlargement (iodine-deficiency goiter), the obvious sign of which is swelling in the neck.

(ii) Hypothyroidism.

Q.41. Name the goitrogenic foods?

Ans. (i) Cauliflower

(ii) Broccoli (a variety of cauliflower with greenish flower head)

(iii) Cabbage, etc.

Q.42. What happens in hypothyroidism?

Ans. In hypothyroidism, the child becomes a dwarf or cretin. A cretin grows slowly (stunted growth) and has a low mentality (low IQ); his hair are scanty and coarse and skin is thick and dry. His BMR is also low.

Q.43 What is myxoedema?

Ans. If the thyroid gland is removed or it becomes subnormal in activity in the adults then myxoedema develops in which :

(i) the skin becomes thick and dry.

(ii) the hair become coarser and fallout.

(iii) there is disinclination towards work, either physically or mentally.

(iv) there is a tendency to put on weight.

(v) the metabolic rate is reduced, nitrogen metabolism gets lowered and the body's temperature is subnormal.

(vi) Ossification of the bones gets delayed.

Q.44. What is hyperthyroidism?

Ans. (i) It's state in which thyroid gland is too active as a result of which a condition known as exophthalmic goiter occurs.

(ii) A common symptom of this disease is the building of the eyes.

(iii) This disease is also known as **'Graves'** or **Basedow's'** disease.

(iv) The BMR is high.

(v) Nitrogen metabolism gets increased.

(vi) Hair are fine.

(vii) The body's temperature remains above the normal.

(viii) The patient is nervous and irritable

(ix) His IQ is above than normal

(x) He or she is underweight

(xi) His/her heart beats are generally faster and irregular.

Q.45. Name the sources of fluorine.

Ans. (i) Drinking water

(ii) Tea

(iii) Flesh of marine fishes also contains small amounts.

Q.46. What is the daily requirement of fluorine for adults and children?

Ans. About 1 part of fluorine in one million parts of drinking water (1 PPM) is OK for both i.e., adults and children.

Q.47. What are the main functions of fluorine?

Ans. (i) It plays a vital role in the development of tooth and dental health.

(ii) It is also concerned with the development of bones.

Q.48. Whether high concentration of fluorides are toxic to human beings? Which disease is caused due to high intake of it?

Ans. (i) Yes, **Dental fluorosis (mottled enamel)** is caused in the children.

(ii) Hypercalcification of the bone of spine, pelvis and limbs. Its severity is fatal and may cause neurological disturbances as a result of which such individuals may become crippled.

Q.49. What are the general functions of minerals?

Ans. (i) As structural components of body tissues.
(ii) In the maintenance of acid-base balance.
(iii) In the regulation of body fluids.
(iv) In the transport of gases.
(v) In the contraction of muscles.

Q.50. Name the conditions in which serum potassium level gets increased?

Ans. (i) Addison's disease
(ii) Diabetic acidosis
(iii) Chronic renal disease
(iv) Shock.

Q.51. Name the conditions in which serum potassium level gets decreased.

Ans. (i) Diarrhoea
(ii) Metabolic alkalosis
(iii) Familial periodic paralysis.

Q.52. Name the conditions in which serum sodium level gets increased.

Ans. (i) Cushing's disease
(ii) Excessive sweating.

Q.53. Name the conditions in which serum sodium level gets decreased.

Ans. (i) Vomiting
(ii) Diarrhoea
(iii) Acute Addison's disease
(iv) Nephrosis
(v) Intestinal obstruction (vi) Severe burns.

Q.54. What is the daily requirement of calcium for adults, pregnant or lactating women, infants/children?

Ans. 800 mg, 1.2 g and 0.4-1.2 g respectively.

Q.55. Name the calcium rich-foods.

(i) Dairy products like milk, cheese, khoa, curd, hard water, lime used with betel leaves.
(ii) Dark green leafy vegetables like radish-tops etc., carrot, soyabean, drybeans, etc.
(iii) Egg-yolk.

Q.56. Name the conditions in which serum calcium level is increased.

Ans. (i) Hyperparathyroidism
(ii) Hypervitaminosis-D.

Q.57. Name the conditions in which serum calcium level gets decreased.

Ans. (i) Hypothyroidism
(ii) Increased loss of calcium due to kidney diseases
(iii) Decreased absorption from the intestines
(iv) Decreased dietary intake.

Q.58. Name the factors which affect the absorption of calcium.

Ans. (i) Vitamin D promotes the absorption of calcium.
(ii) High protein diet also promotes the absorption of calcium.
(iii) Absorption of calcium requires acidic pH.
(iv) Oxalates, phosphates and phytates inhibit the absorption of calcium.

Q.59. What is the transported form of iron?

Ans. Transferrin.

Q.60. What is the state of iron in transferrin?

Ans. Ferric form.

Q.61. Name few iron containing compounds.

Ans. (i) Hemoglobin
(ii) Ferritin
(iii) Transferrin
(iv) Myoglobin
(v) Enzymes like catalase, cytochromes b, c_1, c and a, catalase and peroxidase.

Q.62. What is the daily requirement of iron?

Ans. 15-20 mg.

Q.63. By which 'chemical compound' iron store of liver is known as?

Ans. Ferritin.

Q.64. By which 'Chemical compound' iron store of spleen is known as?

Ans. Ferritin.

Q.65. The deposition of which substance causes haemosiderosis?

Ans. Haemosiderin.

Q.66. What is haemosiderin?

Ans. It's a form of ferritin complexed with other proteins and iron.

Q.67. Which cheating agent has got the capability to induce the excretion of iron to some extent through the kidneys?

Ans. Desferrioxamine.

Q.68. Which vitamin is responsible to increase the absorption of iron strongly?

Ans. Vitamin-C (ascorbic acid)

Q.69. How many subunits does the molecule of ferritin contain?

Ans. 24

Q.70. What is the molecular weight of ferritin?

Ans. 5 lakhs.

Q.71. Name the antioxidant minerals.

Ans. Copper, Manganese, Zinc and selenium.

Q.72. What is the biochemical action of copper?

Ans. Copper is an essential component of a number of proteins (e.g. throcuprein, hepatocuprein) and enzymes (e.g. lysyl hydroxylase, dopamine, β–hydroxylase).

Q.73. What is the biochemical action of manganese?

Ans. Manganese shows a free radical scavenging activity. The chain breaking antioxidant capacity of manganese seems to be related to the rapid quenching of peroxyl radicals.

Q.74. What is the biochemical action of Zinc?

Ans. **Zinc is a cofactor for over 100 enzymes and is important in nucleic acids metabolism and protein synthesis.**

Zinc has been shown to have an antioxidant role in defined chemical systems. Administration of pharmacological doses of zinc *in vivo* has a protective effect against general and liver specific pro-oxidants.

Q.75. What is the biochemical action of selenium?

Ans. Selenium is an essential trace element and is an integral part of the enzyme system glutathione peroxidase, **which protects intracellular structures against oxidative damage**. Selenium is being increasingly recognized as a versatile anticarcinogenic agent.

Q.76 Which mineral is required for the decomposition of hydrogen peroxide?

Ans. Selenium

Q.77 Which mineral is required for the formation of prothrombin?

Ans. Calcium.

Q.78 What is osteoporosis?

Ans. It literally means abnormally porous bones which are compressible like a sponge. This disorder of the skeleton weakans this bones to the tune of frequent fractures (breaks) in the bones.

Q.79 In which two forms, phosphorus remains present in the body?

Ans. (i) Inorganic form, and
(ii) Organic form

Q.80 What is the significance of inorganic phosphorus in humans?

Ans. It is essential for the formation and development of bones and teeth. It helps in ossification and gets deposited as calcium phosphate. It also remains present in soft tissues and various body fluids as sodium and potassium phosphates.

Q.81 What is the significance of organic phosphorus in humans?

Ans. Phosphorus containing organic compounds include:
(i) Phosphorus esters of monosaccharides such as glucose-6-PO_4, dihydroxyacetone phosphate, etc.
(ii) Phospholipids,
(iii) Nucleic acids,
(iv) High energy compounds like ATP, etc. which produce energy.

Q.82 What are the sources of calcium and phosphorus?

Ans. Milk and dairy products are rich sources. Egg yolk, dry fruits, legumes, cabbage and cauliflower are also good sources.

Q.83 What are the biochemical functions of calcium?

Ans.
(i) Calcification of the growing bones and teeth and afterwards maintenance of mature bones.
(ii) It acts as an activator for several enzymes like adenyl cyclase, ATPase and protein kinase, etc.
(iii) It is required for clotting of blood.
(iv) It is also required for contraction of muscles.
(v) It is also required to regulate the permeability of the capillary walls and excitability of the nerve fibers.
(vi) It is required for the secretion of various hormones
(vii) **It also acts as a second messenger.**

Q.84 What are the biochemical functions of phosphorus?

Ans.
(i) Phosphorus along with calcium is very essential for mineralization of bones.
(ii) It plays an important role in the **regulation of acid base balance.**
(iii) **As a component of several coenzymes,** it also participates in various enzyme-catalysed reactions.
(iv) Pi as well as organic esters of phosphoric acid, such as ADP, glucose-6-PO_4 etc. are necessary for the metabolism of carbohydrates, and thus, in the production of energy.

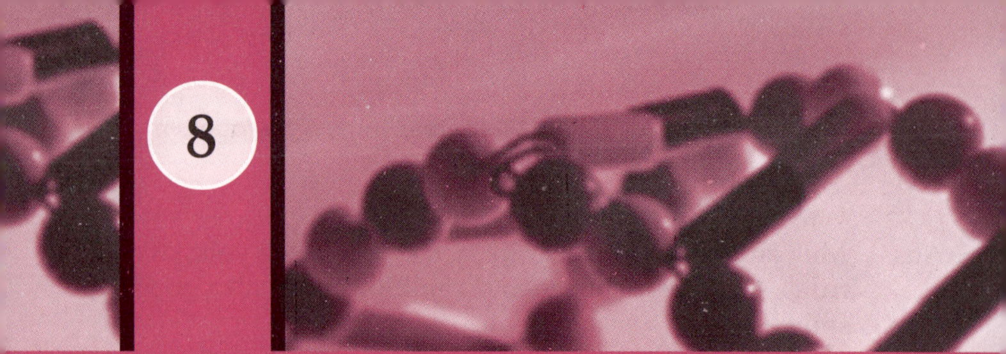

8

Blood

Q.1. What are the main functions of blood?

Ans. (i) As a carrier of oxygen

(ii) As a carrier of metabolic wastes of the body to different organs like kidney, lungs, skin and intestine for their removal

(iii) In the maintenance of acid-base balance

(iv) In the maintenance of the temperature of body

(v) In transporting food materials to the tissues

(vi) In the regulation of water balance

(vii) Defense against infection

(viii) Prevention of haemorrhage

Q.2. What is the pH of blood?

Ans. 7.4 (7.35-7.45)

Q.3. What is the average volume of blood in the body?

Ans. 6-8% of the body weight.

Q.4. What is the colour of blood and why?

Ans. It is red on account of the hemoglobin of erythrocytes.

Q.5. What is the composition of blood?

Ans. (i) Cellular fraction: This fraction contains erythrocytes (red cells), leucocytes (white cells) and platelets

(ii) Plasma fraction (it's colloidal in nature).

Q.6. Name the substance of blood-clot.

Ans. Fibrin.

Q.7. Name the inhibitors of blood coagulation.

Ans. (i) Oxalates
(ii) Citrates
(iii) Heparin.

Q.8. What are the factors which delay coagulation of blood?

Ans. (i) Low level of prothrombin
(ii) Deficiency of vitamin C

Q.9. What is the specific gravity of blood?

Ans. 1.054-1.060

Q.10. What is the mechanism of blood clotting?

Ans. (i) Activation stage :
Prothrombin + thromboplastin + $Ca^{++} \rightarrow$ Thrombin
(ii) Conversion stage :
Fibrinogen + thrombin $\longrightarrow$ Fibrin (clot)

Q.11. What are thromboplastins chemically?

Ans. These are complex lipoproteins in which cephalic or other phospholipids are components.

Q.12. What is hemophilia?

Ans. (i) This is also known as bleeder's disease in which there is either deficiency or absence of antihemophilic globulin i.e. factor VIII in blood.
(ii) This is a congenital disease and is inherited as a sex-linked Mendelian recessive which occurs frequently in males but is transmitted through females.
(iii) The blood of hemophilics generally clots very slowly, and the clots are not normally firm and do not hold well.

Q.13. What is serum?

Ans. The blood on clotting (without any anticoagulant) gives a clear slightly yellowish supernatant which is called serum.

Q.14. What is plasma?

Ans. Plasma is obtained from blood which is prevented from clotting.

Q.15. What is the difference between serum and plasma?

Ans. Serum differs from plasma in that it does not contain fibrinogen.

Q.16. What is the normal level of hemoglobin in blood in males and females respectively?

Ans. (i) 14-18 g% (males)
(ii) 11-16 g% (females).

Q.17. Where does hemoglobin remain present?

Ans. Red blood cells.

Q.18. To which class of proteins hemoglobin belongs?

Ans. It belongs to a class of conjugated protein. It has been put in the category of chromoprotein and metalloprotein as well.

Hemoglobin = Heme + Globin

Q.19. What is the prosthetic group of hemoglobin?

Ans. Heme (a cyclic tetrapyrrole)

Q.20. What it heme?

Ans. Heme is ferrous protoporphyrin

Q.21. What is the state of iron in hemoglobin?

Ans. Iron is present in ferrous state (i.e. + 2 state).

Q.22. What are the salient features of the structure of hemoglobin molecule?

Ans. It contains the following:

(i) 4 iron atoms (in the ferrous state)
(ii) 4 heme groups
(iii) Large proportion of histidine residues, about 35 per molecule
(iv) At least 4 sulfhydryl (-SH) groups
(v) The globin part of Hb is made-up of 4 polypeptide chains, two α- and two β-chains, both types having valine as the N-terminal amino acids.

Q.23. What are the starting materials for the synthesis of hemoglobin?

Ans. Succinyl CoA and glycine.

Q.24. In which state iron remains present in methemoglobin?

Ans Ferric form

Q.25. What is foetal hemoglobin?

Ans. In addition to normal adult hemoglobin (A), it has long been known that a different hemoglobin remains present in the blood of the newly born which has been designated as foetal hemoglobin or hemoglobin F.

Q.26. Which type of hemoglobin remains present in RBCs in sickle cell anemia?

Ans. Hemoglobin S.

Q.27. Of how many polypeptide chains globin molecule is made-up?

Ans. (i) Two polypeptide chains of one kind, and

(ii) Two polypeptide chains of another kind meaning to say, it's a tetramer.

Q.28. How many amino acids are there roughly in each polypeptide chain?

Ans. About 150

Q.29. What is abnormal hemoglobin?

Ans. The substitution of any one of these amino acids by another results in the formation of an abnormal chain and so of an abnormal hemoglobin.

Q.30. Which amino acid of normal hemoglobin is replaced by which amino acid and at which position in sickle cell anemia i.e., HbS?

Ans. In the β-chain of normal hemoglobin, the sixth amino acid from the *N*-terminal is glutamic acid which in case of HbS is replaced by valine.

Q.31. How many types of abnormal hemoglobins known today, name some of them?

Ans. More than 200 types are known today, examples are

(i) Hemoglobin-S
(ii) Hemoglobin-H
(iii) Hemoglobin-C
(iv) Hemoglobin-E
(v) Hemoglobin-M
(vi) Hemoglobin-G Honolulu
(vii) Hemoglobin-M Saskatoon
(viii) Hemoglobin-O Indonesia
(ix) Hemoglobin-D Punjab, etc.

Q.32. What is porphyria?

Ans. Accumulation of coproporphyrin and uroporphyrin in the blood with the excessive elimination in urine and faeces is called porphyria.

Q.33. What is thalassemia?

Ans. Thalassemias are characterized by defects in the synthesis of hemoglobin subunits, and so β-thalassemia results when there is insufficient production of β-globin.

In α-thalassemia, there is a corresponding suppression in the synthesis of α-globin.

Q.34. Name the important buffers of the blood.

Ans. (i) Bicarbonate buffer, CO_2/HCO_3^-

(ii) Hemoglobin buffer, HHb/Hb- and $HHbO_2/HbO_2^-$

(iii) Protein buffer, H-protein/Protein$^-$

(iv) Phosphate buffer, $H_2PO_4^-/HPO_4^-$

Q.35. For what the abbreviation HbS stands?

Ans. Sickle cell hemoglobin

Q.36. What are the subunits in HbS?

Ans. ααββ

Q.37. What are the changes in the amino acids in case of HbS?

Ans. Glutamic acid is replaced by valine at the 6th position of β–chain.

Q.38. What is the clinical manifestation of sickle cell anaemia?

Ans. Haemolytic anaemia

Q.39. For what HbH stands?

Ans. α–thalassemia

Q.40. What are the subunits of α-thalassemia?

Ans. ββββ

Q.41. What is the abnormality of α-thalassemia?

Ans. Defective synthesis of α-chains

Q.42. What is the clinical manifestation of α-thalassemia?

Ans. Mild anaemia

Q.43. What are the subunits of β-thalassemia?

Ans. ααγγ

Q.44. What is the abnormality in β-thalassemia?

Ans. Failure to switch from synthesis of γ-chains to β-chains at birth which results in abnormal oxygen affinity.

Q.45. What is the clinical manifestation of β-thalassemia?

Ans. Anaemia

Q.46. For what HbA stands?

Ans. Normal hemoglobin

Q.47. Of how many amino acids each polypeptide chain of hemoglobin is composed?

Ans. About 150

Q.48. What is the exact colour of blood in the arteries?

Ans. Bright red (well oxygenated)

Q.49. What is the exact colour of blood in veins?

Ans. Dark red (less oxygenated)

Q.50. What is the specific gravity of blood?

Ans. 1.045-1.065

Q.51. What is the normal temperature of human body?

Ans. 37°C or 98.6°F

Q.52. What is the full form of EDTA?

Ans. Ethylenediaminetetra-acetic acid.

Q.53. How many times blood is thicker than water?

Ans. 4.5 times

Q.54. What is the volume of blood?

Ans. Its weight is 9% of the body's total weight. (the average man has a blood volume of 5-6 litres, the average woman 4-5 litres).

Q.55. What is the percentage of plasma in blood?

Ans. 55

Q.56. What is the approximate number of red cells per cubic millimeter of blood in the males?

Ans. Approximately 55,00,000

Q.57. What is the approximate number of red cells per cubic millimeter of blood in the females?

Ans. Approximately 48,00,000

Q.58. What is the primary role of erythrocytes?

Ans. To carry molecular oxygen to all cells and the tissues of the body.

Q.59. Name the main ingredient of RBCs which is responsible to carry molecular oxygen to all the cells and tissues of our body.

Ans. Hemoglobin.

Q.60. What do you understand by the term 'hemoglobin'?

Ans. Heme [(hematin (a non-protein portion)] + globin (blood protein)

Q.61. What metal does heme contain?

Ans. Iron

Q.62. How many molecules of hemoglobin are found in one erythrocyte?

Ans. Several millions

Q.63. Name the phenomenon of manufacturing of red blood cells.

Ans. Erythropoiesis

Q.64. By which circulating hormone of blood erythropoiesis gets stimulated?

Ans. Erythropoietin

Q.65. After birth, where does red cell formation take place?

Ans. Red bone marrow

Q.66. What is the life span of RBCs?

Ans. About 120 days

Q.67. Which vitamin is required for complete maturation of RBCs?

Ans. B_{12}

Q.68. The absorption of which vitamin is promoted from the food, we eat, by the intrinsic factor, which is secreted by the inner mucosal lining of the stomach.

Ans. B_{12}

Q.69. What is the life span of WBCs?

Ans. 13-20 days

Q.70. Besides iron and cobalt, which basic metal is essential for RBCs formation.

Ans. Copper.

Q.71 What's anaemia?

Ans. It's an abnormal condition in which blood lacks either its normal number of red cells or its normal concentration of hemoglobin.

Q.72 Some hemolytic anaemias are caused by excessive destruction of which cells?

Ans. RBCs.

Q.73 What is Polycythemia?

Ans. It is characterized by the production of large number of red blood cells than the normal number .

Q.74 What is the main function of WBCs?

Ans. The white cells of the blood (leucocytes) are primarily concerned with the body's defence system against any infection.

Q.75 What is the normal range of leucocytes (TLC)?

Ans. 5,000 - 10,000 cells per cubic millimeter

Q.76 Where are antibodies produced?

Ans. Lymphocytes

Q.77 Where Monocytes are produced?

Ans. Bone-marrow.

Q.78 What is leukopenia?

Ans. A condition in which there is a decrease in the number of total leukocytes (white cells) count.

Q.79 What is the life-span of blood platelets (thrombocytes)?

Ans. Approximately 8 days.

Q.80 Which Vitamin is essential for the synthesis of prothrombin?

Ans. Vitamin K

Q.81 Where are antibodies formed?

Ans. Antibodies (lysine, opsonin, agglutinins and antitoxins) are formed by the reticuloendothelial system (spleen, liver, lymph nodes, and bone marrow).

Q.82 What is the range of pH of blood?

Ans. 7.35 to 7.45 (average 7.4)

Q.83 What is the major purpose of blood buffer system?

Ans. To maintain acid–base balance

Q.84 Name the most important buffer system of human body.

Ans. Bicarbonate.

Q.85 Name the other two important buffer systems of human body which are less important than the bicarbonate buffer.

Ans. Phosphate buffer system and the protein buffer system.

Q.86 How the bicarbonate buffer system is denoted (write the exact chemical formula)?

Ans. $NaHCO_3$ — H_2CO_3

Q.87 How the phosphate buffer system is denoted (write the exact chemical formula)?

Ans. NaH_3PO_4 — Na_2HPO_4

Q.88 What is thrombus?

Ans. The formation of a blood clot is called thrombus.

Q.89 Which enzyme is liberated from the disintegrated blood platelets?

Ans. Thromboplastinogenase.

Q.90 In which organ, heparin is produced?

Ans. Liver

Q.91 Name the anticoagulant polysaccharide?

Ans. Heparin

Q.92 What is embolism?

Ans. It is the blocking of vessels/arteries by an object (embolus) that has been carried by the blood stream from another site.

Q.93 What is purpura?

Ans. It is a bleeding disorder in which hemorrhages occur in the skin and mucous membranes.

Q.94 What is the normal prothrombin time?

Ans. 15-20 seconds

Q.95 What is anaphylactic shock?

Ans. It is a massive response to an allergen which is caused when a drug or vaccine or any allergen to which a person is sensitive, has entered the circulatory system.

Q.96 By what other name 'denatured hemoglobin' is known?

Ans. Heinz Bodies

Q.97. What are T and R forms of hemoglobin?

Ans (i) **T-form of Hb :** The deoxy form of Hb exists in a T or taut (tense) form. T-form has low affinity for oxygen.

(ii) **R-form of Hb :** The binding of oxygen destabilizes Hb structure to result in relaxed form (R-form). This form has high affinity for oxygen.

Q.98. What do you know about the structure of hemoglobin?

Ans. It's a conjugated protein having a molecular weight of 64,450 containing globin–the protein part and the heme- the non-protein part (prosthetic group). The globin is composed of 2α and 2β chains. Hence, contains protoporphyrin IX (with 4 pyrrole rings) with iron in the centre.

Q.99. What are the different types of hemoglobins?

Ans. In adults, about 95% is hemoglobin A_1 (with 2α and 2β chains) and rest 5% hemoglobin A_2 (with 2α and 2δ chains). Fetal hemoglobin (with 2α and 2γ chains) is synthesized during fetal development and a little of it may be found in adults. **Increase in glycosylated hemoglobin (>5%) is observed in the patients of diabetes mellitus.**

Q.100. What is methemoglobin?

Ans. Hemoglobin (Fe^{2+}) can be oxidized to methemoglobin (Fe^{3+}) by certain agents like H_2O_2, free radicals, drugs, etc. Methemoglobin is unable to bind to oxygen.

Q.101. What are hemoglobinopathies?

Ans. These are the disorders caused by the synthesis of abnormal hemoglobin molecules or the production of insufficient amount of normal hemoglobin or rarely both, for instance sickle cell anemia, HbC, HbD, HbE, HbG, HbH, HbI, HbM, etc. **(today more than 200 abnormal hemoglobins are known).**

Q.102. What is sickle cell anemia?

Ans. Sickle cell anemia (Hb S) is the most common form of

abnormal hemoglobins. **Red blood cells of such patients adopt shape of a sickle, hence called as sickle cell anemia.** In this type, glutamate at the 6th position of β chain is replaced by valine (Glu β 6 $\longrightarrow$ Val). Hbs, is found to be associated with many disorders like:

(i) Hemolytic anemia
(ii) Increased susceptibility to infections
(iii) Tissue damage, and
(iv) Premature death

Q.103. What do you know about thalassemias?

Ans. Thalassemias are a group of disorders characterized by impairement/imbalance in the synthesis of globin (α or β) chains of Hb e.g., α–thalassemia, β-thalassemia.

Q.104. What are porphyrins?

Ans. These are the cyclic compounds made-up of four pyrrole rings held together.

Heme is an iron-containing porphyrin while chlorophyll is a magnesium containing porphyrin.

Q.105. What are porphyrias?

Ans. These are the metabolic disorders of heme synthesis characterized by the increased excretion of porphyrins, or porphyrin precursors, e.g., acute intermittent porphyria (enzyme defect **uroporphyrinogen-I synthase**); congenital erythropoietic porphyria (enzyme **defect uroporphyrinogen-II cosynthase); variegate porphyria (enzyme defect–protoporphyrinogen oxidase).**

Q.106. Name the requirement of haemopoitic factors.

Ans. (a) Iron
(b) Folic acid and
(c) Vitamin B_{12}.

Q.107. By which technique serum ferritin and serum transferrin receptor are determined?

Ans. ELISA

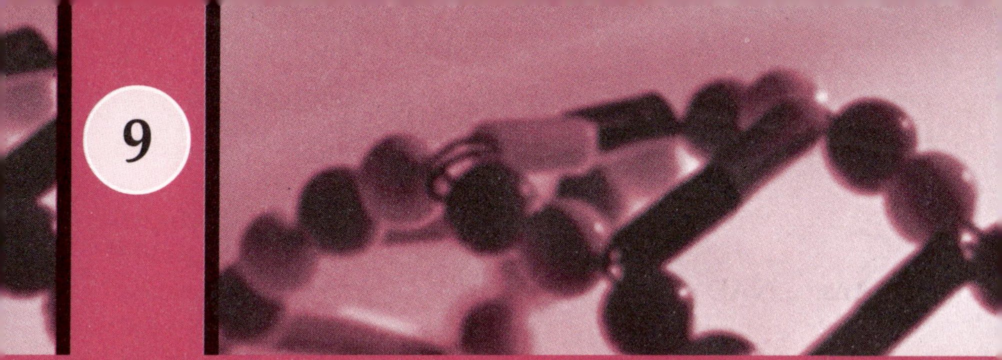

9

ENZYMES

Q.1. What are enzymes?

Ans. (i) These are organic compounds
(ii) They act as biological catalysts
(iii) All enzymes are proteinous in nature
(iv) These are naturally occurring substances which are colloidal in nature.

Q.2. What is a substrate?

Ans. A substance on which enzyme acts is called a substrate.

Q.3. What is a coenzyme or prosthetic group? What is an apoenzyme? What is a holoenzyme?

Ans. It is a thermolabile non-proteinous part which remains closely associated with the enzyme protein and may take part in the enzyme action. Usually such a non-proteinous molecule is called a coenzyme or prosthetic group.

The protein part of such an enzyme is called an apoenzyme and the composite enzyme molecule i.e. (apoenzyme + coenzyme) is called holoenzyme.

Q.4. Give some examples of coenzymes.

Ans. (i) NAD^+
(ii) $NADP^+$
(iii) FAD
(iv) TPP
(v) Pyridoxal phosphate
(vi) ATP
(vii) Coenzyme A, etc.

Q.5. Which coenzyme is required by the enzymes lactic dehydrogenase and alcohol dehydrogenase?

Ans. NAD^+

Q.6. What are the full forms of NAD^+, $NADP^+$, FAD, TPP, FMN and ATP?

Ans. (i) Nicotinamide adenine dinucleotide
(ii) Nicotinamide adenine dinucleotide phosphate
(iii) Flavin adenine dinucleotide
(iv) Thiamine pyrophosphate
(v) Flavin mono nucleotide
(vi) Adenosine triphosphate

Q.7. What is the name of coenzyme 'Q'?

Ans. Ubiquinone.

Q.8. Which coenzyme participates in the respiratory chain?

Ans. Coenzyme 'Q' i.e. ubiquinone.

Q.9. Which coenzyme is required by the enzymes glucose-6-P-dehydrogenase and 6-phosphogluconate dehydrogenase?

Ans. $NADP^+$.

Q.10. Which coenzyme is required by the enzyme succinic dehydrogenase?

Ans. FAD

Q.11. Name the coenzyme which is required by transaminases.

Ans. Pyridoxal phosphate

Q.12. Which coenzyme is required by hexokinases?

Ans. ATP

Q.13. What is the full form of Km?

Ans. Michaelis constant

Q.14. Define Km.

Ans. It is the substrate concentration (in moles per litre) at which half of the maximum velocity is obtained.

Q.15. What are the main types of inhibition?

Ans. (a) Competitive inhibition
(b) Non-competitive inhibition

Q.16. What is competitive inhibition?

Ans. In this type, the inhibitor bears a close structural similarity to the real substrate of the enzyme and competes with the substrate for occupying the binding site of the enzyme molecule.

Q.17. Give important examples of lyases.

Ans. Fumarase which converts fumaric acid into malic acid.

Q.18. Give important examples of competitive inhibitors.

Ans. They include the inhibition of :

(i) succinic dehydrogenase (substrate is succinate) by malonate

(ii) lactate dehydrogenase (substrate is lactate) by oxalate

(iii) aconitase (substrate is citrate) by fluorocitrate

(iv) monoamine oxidase (substrate is monoamines) by monoguanidines.

Q.19. Name the substrate and competitive inhibitor of succinic dehydrogenase.

Ans. Succinic acid (substrate) and malonic acid (substrate-analogue inhibitor)

Q.20. What is non-competitive inhibition?

Ans. In this type, the inhibitor has no structural similarity with the substrate, therefore, it does not compete with the substrate for occupying binding site of the enzyme.

Q.21. Give some important examples of non-competitive inhibition.

Ans. They include the inhibitors of:

(i) Acetylcholine esterase
(ii) Trypsin
(iii) Chymotrypsin
} by Diisopropyl-fluorophosphate

Q.22. What is the classification of enzymes?

Ans. (i) Oxidoreductases

(ii) Transferases

(iii) Hydrolases

(iv) Lyases

(v) Isomerases, and

(vi) Ligases.

Q.23. Give important examples of oxidoreductases.

Ans. (i) Xanthine oxidase which converts xanthine into uric acid

(ii) Cytochrome oxidase which converts reduced cytochrome C into oxidized cytochrome C

Q.24. Give important example of transferases.

Ans. Glucokinase that acts in the following manner:

$$\text{Glucose} + \text{ATP} \longrightarrow \text{Glucose-6-}PO_4 + \text{ADP}$$

Q.25. Give important example of hydrolases.

Ans. (i) Pepsin which converts proteins into peptones

(ii) α-amylase which converts starch into dextrins

(iii) Glucose-6-phosphatase which converts glucose-6-PO_4 into glucose

Q.26. Give important examples of isomerases.

Ans. (i) Triose phosphate isomerase which converts glyceraldehyde-3-phosphate into dihydroxyacetone phosphate.

(ii) UDP-glucose epimerase which converts UDP-glucose into UDP-galactose.

Q.27. Give important examples of ligases.

Ans. (i) Pyruvate carboxylase which converts pyruvate into oxaloacetate.

(ii) Glutamine synthetase which converts L-glutamate into L-glutamine.

Q.28. Where are the enzymes for the following, remain located in the cell?

(i) Glycolysis

(ii) Glycogenesis

(iii) Fatty acid synthesis

(iv) HMP shunt

(v) Catabolism of purines and pyrimidines

Ans. In the extra-mitochondrial fraction of cytoplasm (cytosol).

Q.29. What is the difference between prosthetic group and coenzyme?

Ans. Prosthetic group remains tightly bound to the enzyme whereas coenzymes exist in the solution in free state and contact the enzyme only at the site of reaction.

Q.30. Where are the enzymes for the following remain located in the cell?
(i) Electron transport chain (ETC)
(ii) Respiratory chain
(iii) Oxidative phosphorylation

Ans. In the inner membrane of the mitochondria.

Q.31. Where are the enzymes for the following remain located in the cell?
(i) TCA-cycle
(ii) β-oxidation of fatty acids
(iii) Urea synthesis

Ans. In the fluid matrix of the mitochondria.

Q.32. What is an allosteric site?

Ans. Site other than the active site is called as the allosteric site.

Q.33. What is feed back inhibition?

Ans. This refers to the inhibition of the activity of an enzyme in a biosynthetic pathway by an end product of that pathway which may be represented by the following equation :

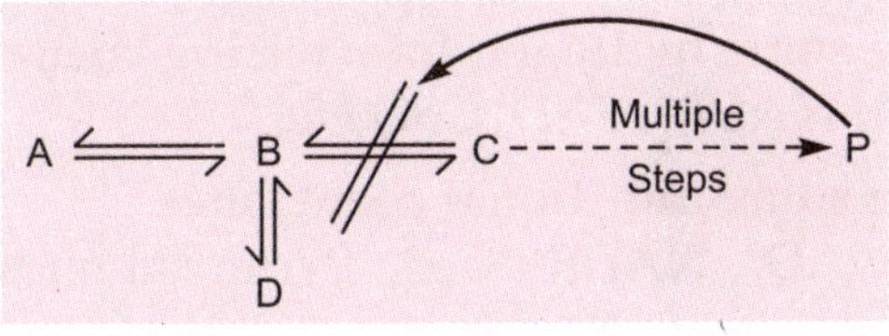

Q.34. What are antienzymes?

Ans. These are the substances produced in the serum as a result of repeated injection of certain enzymes which prevent the normal action of the enzyme injected.

Q.35. Give an example of feed back inhibition.

Ans. Cholesterol inhibits its own synthesis in the liver by inhibiting the enzyme HMG-CoA reductase.

Q.36. Name two enzymes which are used as a medicine to dissolve thrombus (clots)?

Ans. (i) Streptokinase
(ii) Urokinase

Q.37. What are constitutive enzymes?

Ans. Constitutive enzymes are those enzymes which remain virtually present at a constant concentration during the life of a cell.

Q.38. What is the commercial source of urokinase?

Ans. It is prepared from human urine.

Q.39. What is the commercial source of streptokinase?

Ans. It is a bacterial enzyme obtained principally from β-Hemolytic streptococci.

Q.40. What is the commercial source of enzyme hyaluronidase and what is its clinical application?

Ans. It's prepared from mammalian testes. It acts by depolymerizing hyaluronic acid and increasing tissue permeability. It is used in the treatment of traumatic or postoperative edema.

Q.41. What are cofactors?

Ans. The metallic ions which are involved in enzyme activity, e.g. Ca^{++}, Mg^{++}, Mn^{++}, Fe^{++} etc.

Q.42. Name some group transferring coenzymes.

Ans. ATP, Pyridoxal phosphate, CoA etc.

Q.43. Name some hydrogen transferring coenzymes.

Ans. NAD^+, $NADP^+$, FAD, CoQ etc.

Q.44. Name some nutritional coenzymes.

Ans. TPP, NAD^+, $NADP^+$, CoA, Pyridoxal phosphate, etc.

Q.45. What is holoenzyme?

Ans. Apoenzyme + coenzyme = Holoenzyme
(Protein part) (Non-protein part)

Q.46. Name the coenzyme of pyruvate dehydrogenase.

Ans. Thiamine pyrophosphate (TPP).

Q.47. Name the enzyme that was isolated for the first time, crystallized and identified as a protein and by whom.

Ans. Urease by scientist Sumner.

Q.48. What are intracellular and extracellular enzymes?

Ans. Intracellular enzymes are functional within the cells where they are synthesized (e.g., enzymes of TCA cycle) while extracellular are active outside the cells (digestive enzymes of gastrointestinal tract).

Q.49. Name some non-vitamin coenzymes.

Ans. ATP, UDP, CTP, etc.

Q.50. What do you understand by nucleotide coenzymes?

Ans. Some of the coenzymes possess a nitrogenous base, a sugar and phosphate. These are called as nucleotide coenzymes, e.g., NAD^+, $NADP^+$, FMN, FAD, Coenzyme A, UDPG, etc.

Q.51. What do you understand by feed back regulation?

Ans. The process of inhibiting the first step by the final product (end product) in a series of enzyme-catalysed reactions of a metabolic pathway is referred to as feed back regulation.

Q.52. What are proenzymes?

Ans. Some enzymes are synthesized in an inactive form which are referred to as proenzymes (or zymogens). They undergo irreversible changes to produce active enzymes, e.g., proenzymes, namely pepsinogen and chymotrypsinogen are respectively converted to pepsin and chymotrypsin.

Q.53. What do you understand by constitutive enzymes?

Ans. Constitutive (house-keeping) enzymes are the group of enzymes whose synthesis is not controlled and their concentrations do remain fairly constant, e.g. the enzymes of Krebs cycle (TCA cycle).

Q.54. What do you understand by SI unit in enzymes?

Ans. One system international (SI) unit or one International Unit (IU) refers to the activity of the enzymes that catalyses the conversion of one micromole of the substrate per minute.

Q.55. What are ribozymes?

Ans. The RNAs that can function as enzymes are referred to as ribozymes. They are, thus, non-protein enzymes.

Q.56. Give some examples of enzymes used as therapeutic agents.

Ans. (a) Streptokinase is used for dissolving (disintegrating) blood clots.

(b) Asparaginase is used in the treatment of leukaemias.

Q.57. What do you understand by immobilized enzymes?

Ans. Certain enzymes can be made to bind to insoluble inorganic matrix (e.g. cyanogen bromide activated sepharose) to preserve their catalytic activity for long periods. Such enzymes are referred to as immobilized enzymes.

Q.58. What are plasma functional enzymes?

Ans. Certain enzymes normally present in the plasma perform specific functions and are referred to as plasma functional enzymes which include plasmic, choline esterase, lipoprotein lipase, etc.

Q.59. What are plasma non-functional enzymes and what is their importance?

Ans. These enzymes are either found to be totally absent in plasma or in a very low concentration as compared to their levels found in tissues. Estimation of plasma non-functional enzymes is of significance in the diagnosis and prognosis of certain diseases.

Q.60. What is Schardinger's enzyme? What is its common source?

Ans. Xanthine dehydrogenase; Milk.

Q.61. What is the therapeutic use of enzyme hyaluronidase?

Ans. In ophthalmology and dermatology (in the treatment of complications from hyaluronic acid dermal fillers).

10

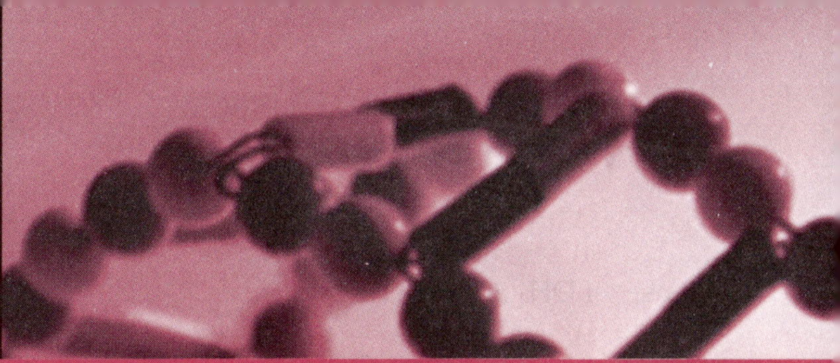

ISOENZYMES

Q.1. What is the difference between isoenzymes or isozymes?

Ans. No difference.

Q.2. What are isoenzymes?

Ans. Isoenzymes are the multiple forms of the same enzyme which may be separated from each other either by electrophoresis or column chromatography. They possess same catalytic activity but differ from each other chemically, immunologically and electrophoretically.

Q.3. Give four important examples of isoenzymes.

Ans. (i) Lactic dehydrogenase
(ii) Creatine phosphokinase
(iii) Glucose-6-phosphate dehydrogenase
(iv) Hexokinase

Q.4. For what abbreviations LDH, CK and CPK stand?

Ans. (i) Lactic dehydrogenase
(ii) Creatine kinase
(iii) Creatine phosphokinase

Q.5. What is the difference between CK and CPK?

Ans. No difference.

Q.6. By which technique isoenzymes of an enzyme are separated from each other?

Ans. Electrophoresis or column chromatography.

Q.7. Which isoenzymes of lactic dehydrogenase are raised in MI?

Ans. LDH_1 and LDH_2.

Q.8. Which enzymes are of diagnostic value in cases of myocardial infarction?

Ans. (i) SGOT (serum glutamic oxaloacetic transaminase) i.e., AST
(ii) CPK (creatine phosphokinase)
(iii) LDH (lactic dehydrogenase)
(iv) HBD (hydroxy butyric dehydrogenase)

Q.9. What is the normal level of SGOT?

Ans. 4-17 IU/l or 8-40 units/ml

Q.10. After how many hours of onset of MI SGOT level in blood is raised and for how long it remains raised?

Ans. The increase begins 3-9 hours after the onset of the attack and returns to normal in 3-8 days. The highest value is found on an average at about 24 hours after the onset

Q.11. What is the normal level of LDH in serum?

Ans. 230-460 IU/l.

Q.12. How long the level of LDH in blood remains raised in blood after an attack of MI?

Ans. It may last as long as 14 days.

Q.13. In which disorders LDH_4 and LDH_5 are raised?

Ans. Liver disorders.

Q.14. Name the isoenzymes of lactate dehydrogenase.

Ans.

LDH_1	HHHH (H_4)
LDH_2	HHHM (H_3M)
LDH_3	HHMM (H_2M_2)
LDH_4	HMMM (HM_3)
LDH_5	MMMM (M_4)

Q.15. Which isoenzyme of CK (CPK) is raised in myocardial infarction?

Ans. CK-MB.

Q.16. When does CK (CPK) start rising in blood after an attack of MI and for how long it remains elevated in blood?

Ans. It increases rapidly within 3-5 hours after the onset of MI and remains elevated in blood for 2-3 days.

Q.17. What is the normal level of CK (CPK) in blood?

Ans. (i) 20-50 IU/l (men)
(ii) 10-37 IU/l (women)

Q.18. What is the usual level of CK (CPK) in muscular dystrophies and dermatomyositis?

Ans. It is usually around 1,000 IU/l.

Q.19. What is the usual level of CK (CPK) in Deuchenne type of muscular dystrophies?

Ans. It is around 10,000 IU/l.

Q.20. What do you know about diagnostic importance of CK (CPK) and its isoenzymes?

Ans. When the total CPK (CK) level is very high, it most often means there has been injury or stress to muscle tissue, the **heart** or the **brain.**

Muscle tissue injury is most likely. When a muscle is damaged, CK leaks into the blood stream. Finding of which specific form of CK is high, helps determine which tissue has been damaged.

The pattern and timing of a rise or fall in CK levels can be significant in making a diagnosis. This is particularly true if a heart attack is suspected.

Most heart attacks are caused by a blood clot that blocks one of the coronary arteries. The coronary arteries bring blood and oxygen to the heart. If the blood flow is blocked, the heart is starved of oxygen and heart cells die. The medical term for this is **myocardial infarction.**

The normal level of CK-MB is 3-5% of toal CK, but peak CK-MB level can range from 15-30% of total CK in post-myocardial infarction.

Isoenzymes of CK : There are three isoenzymes of CK which are as follows:

(i) CK_1 (BB)	:	Brain
(ii) CK_2 (MB)	:	Heart
(iii) CK_3 (MM)	:	Skeletal muscles.

Sl. No.	Isoenzyme	Diagnostic significance	Electrophoretic mobility	Tissue(s) of origin	Mean percentage in blood
1.	BB (CK_1)	Gets raised in brain cancer, brain injury, pulmonary infarction and seizure	Maximum	Brain	0%
2.	MB (CK_2)	Gets raised in heart attack i.e., heart injury, i.e., **Myocardial infarction** within 3-6 hours of MI; peak values reach between 16 and 30 hours; CK-MB returns to normal by 24-36 hours.	Intermediate	Heart muscle	15-30%
3.	MM (CK_3)	Gets raised in muscle diseases (dystrophies, dermatomyositis, polymyositis), after severe exercise and injury to skeletal muscle	Least	Skeletal muscle and heart muscle	70-85%

Q.21. Which reaction is catalysed by CK?

Ans. Following reversible reaction is catalysed :

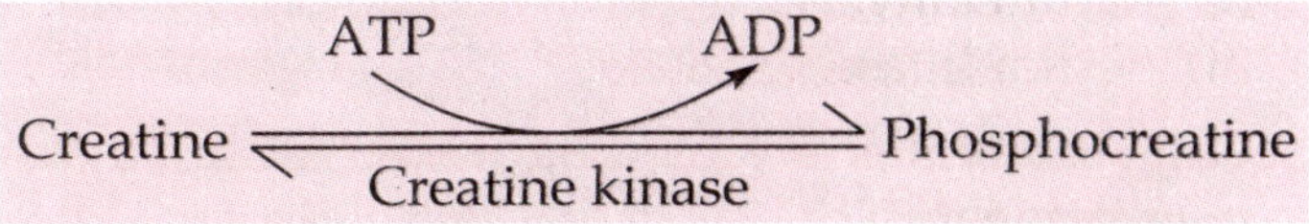

Q.22. How many isoenzymes of hyaluronidase known today?

Ans. Five

Q.23. Whether the estimation of enzyme aldolase or CPK has got much significance in the diagnosis of muscle diseases.

Ans. CPK is more sensitive. These days, estimation of aldolase has been replaced by serum CPK which is more sensitive and more specific as far as diagnosis of muscle diseases is concerned.

Q.24. In what way isoenzymes of alkaline phosphatase are of diagnostic value?

Ans. They throw light as to whether it is a case of bone disease or other diseases like obstructive jaundice.

Q.25. What is the normal level of serum alkaline phosphatase?

Ans. 4-11 King Armstrong units or 60-160 IU/l.

Q.26. How many isoenzymes of $NADP^+$ dependent isocitrate dehydrogenase (ICD or ICDH) are known?

Ans. (i) ICD_1
(ii) ICD_2
(iii) ICD_3
(iv) ICD_4

Q.27. In which disorders, level of isocitrate dehydrogenase is raised in blood?

Ans. In inflammatory, malignant and toxic liver diseases.

Q.28. Name the enzymes which are of diagnostic value in various disorders.

Ans. (i) Alkaline phosphatase
(ii) Glutamic pyruvic transaminase (GPT)
(iii) ICDH (iv) LDH_4 and LDH_5

Q.29. Which enzymes are of diagnostic value in pancreatic diseases?

Ans. (i) Serum amylase
(ii) Serum lipase

Q.30. Which enzymes are of diagnostic value in primary myopathies?

Ans. (i) Aldolase (ii) CPK

Q.31. What are enzyme activators?

Ans. Many enzymes exhibit a specific requirement for a particular ion. These metal ions are called as activators like Mg^{++}, Cu^{++}, Ca^{++}, Mn^{++} etc.

Q.32. What is the diagnostic significance of the measurement of Angiotensin-Converting Enzyme(ACE) in serum?

Ans. It gets elevated in :
(a) Sarcoidosis,
(b) Histoplasmosis,
(c) Alcoholic cirrhosis
(d) Asbestosis,
(e) Amyloidosis,
(f) Hodgkin's disease, and
(g) Silicosis.

Q.33. Name other cardiac markers besides AST, CPK and LDH.

Ans. (a) Troponin - T (cTn T), (b) Troponin - I (cTn I),
(c) Homocysteine, and (d) Myoglobin

Q.34. What are the reliable markers of ventricular function?

Ans. Patients with congestive heart failure have high plasma levels of **Atrial natriuretic peptide (ANP)** and **Brain natriuretic peptide (BNP).**

Q.35. What is the diagnostic significance of C-reactive protein (CRP)?

Ans. It gets elevated in plasma after MI, trauma, neoplastic proliferation, etc.

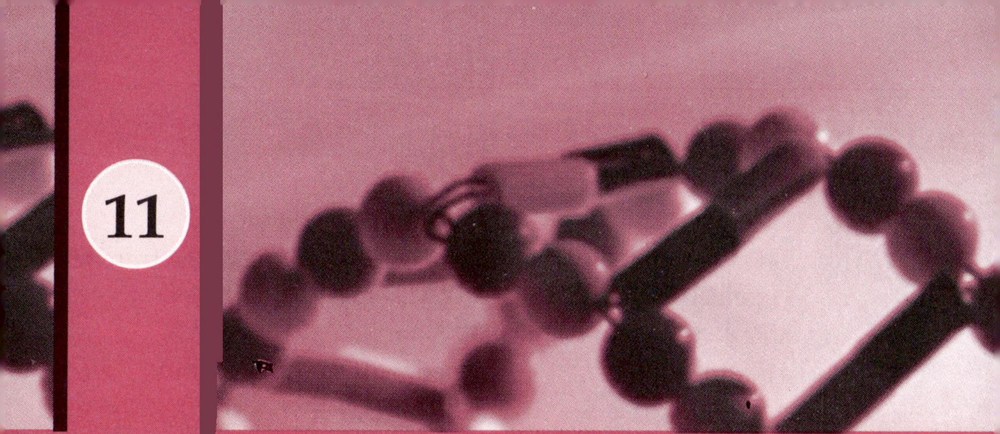

11

BIOLOGICAL OXIDATION

Q.1. What is oxidation?

Ans. It is defined as loss of electrons

$Fe^{++} \longrightarrow Fe^{+++}$ or

removal of hydrogen

$C_2H_5OH \longrightarrow CH_3\ CHO$ or

addition of oxygen to a substance

$CH_3CHO \longrightarrow CH_3\ COOH$

Q.2. What do you mean by biological oxidation?

Ans. The stepwise degradation of metabolite for the liberation of energy (i.e. ATP) carried out in the system is called biological oxidation.

Q.3. Name the components of respiratory chain.

Ans. $NAD^+ \rightarrow Fp \rightarrow CoQ \rightarrow Cyt\ b \rightarrow Cyt\ c_1 \rightarrow Cyt\ c \rightarrow Cyt\ a \rightarrow Cyt\ a_3$

Q.4. Where is ATP utilized?

Ans. (i) Synthetic reactions

(ii) Muscular contraction

(iii) Nerve conduction

(iv) Active transport, etc.

Q.5. What is phosphorylation?

Ans. Formation of ATP (adenosine triphosphate) from ADP and inorganic phosphate is called as phosphorylation.

Q.6. What is oxidative phosphorylation?

Ans. It is a process in which ATP is formed due to the transfer of electron from reduced NAD or reduced FAD to oxygen by a series of electron carriers.

Q.7. Name different enzymes associated with oxidation.

Ans. (i) Oxidases
(ii) Oxygenases
(iii) Aerobic dehydrogenases
(iv) Anaerobic dehydrogenases
(v) Cytochrome oxidase (cytochrome a_3)

Q.8. Name different coenzymes involved in biological oxidation.

Ans. (i) NAD^+
(ii) $NADP^{++}$
(iii) FMN
(iv) FAD
(v) Electron transferring flavoprotein (ETF)
(vi) Coenzyme Q
(vii) Lipoate

Q.9. What is the other name of coenzyme Q?

Ans. Ubiquinone.

Q.10. Give examples of substrate level phosphorylation.

Ans. Conversion of phosphoenolpyruvate to enolpyruvate during glycolysis or conversion of 1, 3-diphosphoglyceric acid to 3-phosphoglyceric acid during glycolysis or conversion of succinyl CoA to succinic acid during TCA cycle.

Q.11. What is the heat formation of ATP from ADP and Pi?

Ans. It is about 7,400 cals.

Q.12. What are the actual sites of phosphorylation in the respiratory chain?

Ans. They are between:
(i) Fp_1 and Fp_2 (1 ATP)
(ii) Cytochrome b and c_1 (1 ATP), and
(iii) Cytochrome aa_3 and oxygen (1 ATP).

Q.13. Name uncouplers of oxidative phosphorylation.

Ans. (i) Dinitrophenol

(ii) Dinitrocresol
(iii) Pentachlorophenol, etc.

Q.14. Name the mechanisms of oxidative phosphorylation.

Ans. (i) Chemical hypothesis
(ii) Chemiosmotic theory

Q.15. What is substrate level phosphorylation?

Ans. In substrate level phosphorylation, formation of high energy phosphate bond takes place at the substrate level without undergoing into the respiratory chain.

Q.16. What is P/O ratio?

Ans. P/O ratio is defined as the number of inorganic phosphates required to phosphorylate ADP per atom of oxygen consumed.

$$\frac{P}{O} = \frac{\text{Number of Pi required to phosphorylate ADP}}{\text{No. of atom of oxygen consumed}}$$

Q.17. Name few reactions where P/O ratio is three.

Ans. **(a)** Pyruvic acid

↓ Pyruvate dehydrogenase complex

Acetyl CoA (when pyruvic acid enters into TCA cycle)

(b) Isocitric acid

↓ Isocitrate dehydrogenase

Oxalosuccinic acid (TCA cycle)

(c) α-ketoglutaric acid

↓ α-ketoglutaric acid dehydrogenase complex

Succinyl CoA (TCA cycle)

(d) Malic Acid
↓ Malic dehydrogenase
Oxaloacetic acid (TCA cycle)

Q.18. Name few reactions where P/O ratio is two.

Ans. (a) Succinate $\xrightarrow[\text{dehydrogenase}]{\text{Succinic}}$ Fumarate (TCA cycle)

(b) Acyl CoA $\xrightarrow[\text{dehydrogenase}]{\text{Acyl CoA}}$ α,β-unsaturated Acyl CoA (β-oxdn. of fatty acids)

Q.19. Name few high energy phosphate compounds.

Ans. (i) ATP
(ii) ADP
(iii) β-Glycerophosphate
(iv) Inosine triphosphate
(v) Creatine phosphate
(vi) S-adenosyl methionine
(vii) UDPG etc.

Q.20. Name few inhibitors of the respiratory chain.

Ans. (i) Barbiturates such as amobarbital
(ii) Piericidin A
(iii) Rotenone (Fish poison)
(iv) Antimycin A
(v) H_2S
(vi) CO
(vii) Cyanides, etc.

Q.21. In cytochrome P-450 for what (i) P and (ii) 450 stand.

Ans. (i) Pigment and
(ii) Maximum i.e. maximum wavelength of absorption

Q.22. What are free radicals?

Ans. These are highly reactive species that have the potential to oxidize biological molecules, including proteins, lipids and DNA.

Q.23. Does imbalance between oxidative stress and antioxidative defence lead to some diseases?

Ans. It leads to various diseases, namely :

(i) Cardiovascular
(ii) Diabetes
(iii) Cancer
(iv) Inflammatory
(v) Neurological, etc.

Q.24. What are the cheaper sources of antioxidants and what about their servings per day?

Ans. Cheaper sources include atleast five servings of fruits and vegetables each day which we the Indians do not consume normally.

Q.25. Which vitamins and pigments have been included as antioxidants and what are their quantities to be taken per day?

Ans. (i) Vitamin A (5000 I.U.)
(ii) Beta carotene (10 mg)
(iii) Vitamin C (100 mg)
(iv) Vitamin E (25 mg)

Q.26. How do the antioxidant vitamins and pigments function biochemically?

Ans. (i) Vitamin A and β-carotene function synergetically with vitamin E to prevent lipid peroxidation.

(ii) Vitamin C is first line plasma anti-oxidant, strongest reductant and radical scavenger.

(iii) Vitamin E is the nature's most effective chain breaking antioxidant, protects cell membranes from peroxi-dative damage.

Scientific evidences indicate that the three major antioxidants i.e., vitamins C, E and carotenoids play a crucial role in preventing or delaying the onset of major degenerative diseases.

Q.27. Which minerals are believed to help in the working of human antioxidant defence?

Ans. Zinc, Copper, Manganese and Selenium.

Q.28. Is cigarette smoke is rich in free radicals?

Ans. Yes.

Q.29. What is the biochemical action of free radicals in cigarette smokers? What is the solution of that?

Ans. They are believed to induce DNA damage that can be prevented by taking antioxidants.

Q.30. What are high–energy compounds?

Ans. The term high–energy compounds (energy rich compounds) is applied to substances that possess free energy to liberate at least 7 cal/mol at pH 7.0. Examples are:

(i) ATP
(ii) Phosphocreatine
(iii) Phosphoenolpyruvate
(iv) 1, 3 - diphosphoglycerate

Q.31. How is ATP synthesized?

Ans. It can be synthesized by the following two ways:

(i) Oxidative phosphorylation linked with electron transport chain is the main source of ATP synthesis.

(ii) Substrate level phosphorylation involves the direct formation of ATP during substrate oxidation in the metabolism, e.g., phosphoenolpyruvate and 1,3 diphosphoglycerate of glycolysis) and succinyl CoA (of TCA cycle) can, transfer high energy phosphate to ultimately produce ATP.

Q.32. How would you define oxidation and reduction?

Ans. Oxidation is the loss of electrons, whereas reduction is the gain of electrons.

Q.33. What is the significance of brown adipose tissue?

Ans. Certain animals possess a specialized tissue called brown adipose tissue in the upper back and neck portions. The mitochondria of these tissues are rich in electron carriers and are specialized to carry out oxidation uncoupled from oxidative phosphorylation which causes liberation of heat when fat is oxidized in the brown adipose tissue. Thus, the presence of active brown adipose tissue in certain animals is believed to protect them from becoming obese, a very good property.

Q.34. How would you justify that mitochondria are the power houses of cell?

Ans. These are the centres for metabolic oxidative reactions to generate reduced coenzymes (NADH and $FADH_2$) which, in turn, are utilized in ETC to liberate energy in the form of ATP, this is the reason, mitochondria are regarded as the power houses of the cell.

Q.35. What are free radicals?

Ans. Partially reduced species of oxygen are collectively referred to as free radicals which are highly reactive and toxic to the cells. Free radicals have a tendency to cause damage to DNA, proteins and unsaturated lipids. **They have been implicated in ageing, inflammation, cancer, etc.** The cells possess defense mechanisms to minimize

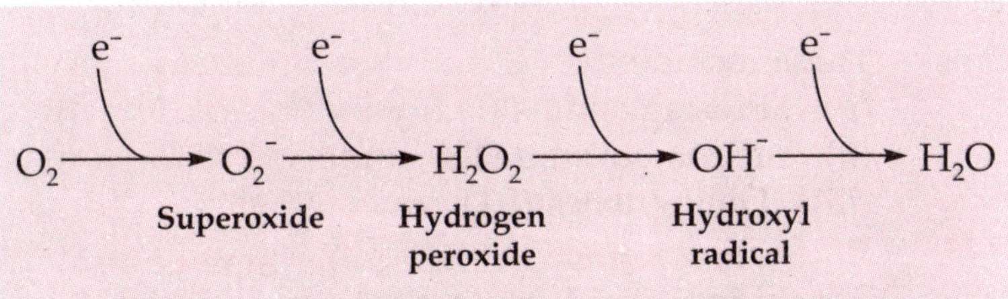

the toxic effects of these compounds. Some enzymes like superoxide dismutase (SOD) and glutathione peroxidase, etc. are of great significance in this regard.

Q.36. What do you know about 'respiratory burst'?

Ans. Free radicals are useful in many ways, for example, in killing microorganisms after phagocytosis (engulfment of bacteria) which is followed by rapid consumption of molecular oxygen that accompanies the formation of superoxide (O_2^-). This process is called as **'respiratory burst'.**

Q.37 The ratio of CO_2 output to O_2 usage is known as:

Ans. Respiratory quotient

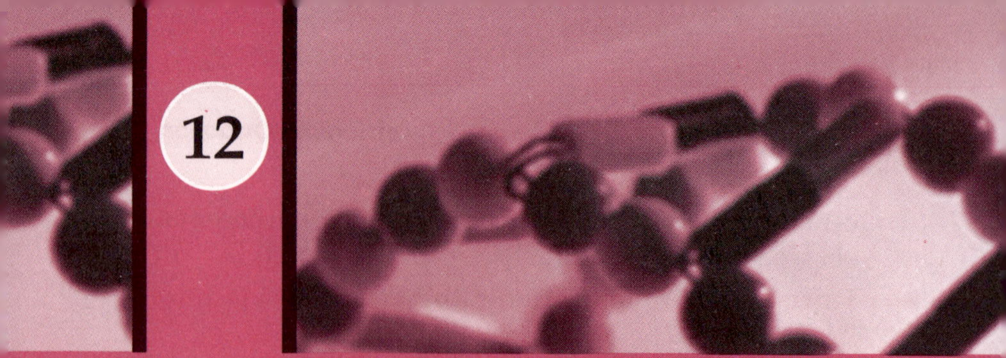

12

EICOSANOIDS (PROSTAGLANDINS) ETC.

Q.1. What are prostaglandins?

Ans. (i) They are **unsaturated cyclic hydroxy fatty acid derivatives** with a five membered ring in a carbon skeleton.

(ii) This **group of hormone like substances** was first of all detected in the seminal fluid of man and other species, hence the name given as prostaglandins.

Q.2. What are eicosanoids?

Ans. These include:

(i) Prostaglandins (PG)

(ii) Thromboxanes (TX), and

(iii) Leukotrienes (LT).

Q.3. What are the precursors of prostaglandins?

Ans. **Arachidonic acid** (**main precursor**), linolenic acid and linoleic acid.

Q.4. What are the various series of prostaglandins?

Ans. A,B,E,F,G,H and I.

Q.5. By the action of which enzyme arachidonic acid is converted into prostaglandins?

Ans. Cyclooxygenase.

Q.6. What are the functions of prostaglandins?

Ans. (i) They help in the fertilization process.

(ii) They are used in the induction of labour at term and also help in the termination of pregnancy.

(iii) They control the secretion of gastric HCl, the excess secretion of which may otherwise cause gastric ulcers.

(iv) These are potent biologically active substances. As little as 1 mg/ml causes contraction of smooth muscle.
(v) They help in preventing conception.
(vi) They control inflammation.
(vii) They give relief in asthma and nasal congestion.
(viii) They control blood pressure.

Q.7. Which prostaglandins are synthesized from linolenic acid?

Ans. PGE_1 and $PGF_{1\alpha}$

Q.8. Which prostaglandins are synthesized from arachidonic acid?

Ans. PGE_2 and $PGF_{2\alpha}$

Q.9. What do you know about thromboxanes?

Ans. (i) These are also C_{20} fatty acid derivatives.
(ii) These are synthesized in platelets.
(iii) They are responsible for vasoconstriction and platelet aggregation.
(iv) They are of different types like TXA, TXB etc.

Q.10. What do you know about leukotrienes?

Ans. (i) These are also C_{20} fatty acid derivatives.
(ii) They are responsible for the causation of vascular permeability.
(iii) They are also responsible for the attraction and activation of leucocytes.
(iv) They appear to be important regulators in many diseases which involve inflammation or immediate hypersensitivity reactions, such as asthma.

Q.11. Who were awarded Nobel Prize for the discovery of Eicosanoids (PGs, thromboxanes, and leukotrienes) and their role in metabolism etc.?

Ans. Bergstrom (Sweden), Samuelsson (Sweden) and Sir John, R (U.K.) were awarded N.P. in Medicine in 1982.

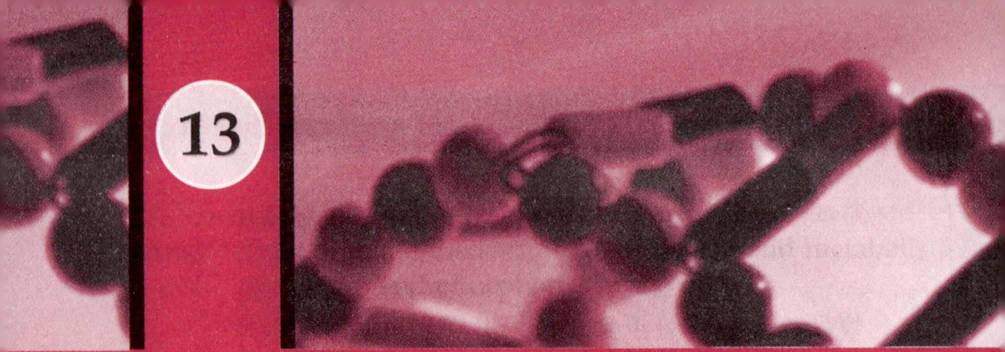

13

VITAMINS

Q.1. What are vitamins?

Ans. Vitamins may be defined **as organic substances** present in naturally occurring foods which are required in small quantity for various physiological processes like maintenance, growth, reproduction etc. of human beings. Besides natural foods, other sources of vitamins include synthetic vitamins, ultraviolet irradiations (precursors of vitamin D), and intestinal microorganisms.

Q.2. What are the types of vitamins?

Ans. Two types:

(i) **Fat soluble vitamins,** and

(ii) **Water soluble vitamins**

Q.3. Name the fat soluble vitamins.

Ans. Vitamins A, D, E and K

Q.4. Name the water soluble vitamins.

Ans. Water soluble vitamins are:

(i) Vitamin B complex group, and

(ii) Vitamin C

Q.5. Name the members of vitamin B complex group.

Ans.

1. Thiamine ($\mathbf{B_1}$),
2. Riboflavin ($\mathbf{B_2}$),
3. Niacin ($\mathbf{B_3}$),
4. Pantothenic acid ($\mathbf{B_5}$),

5. Pyridoxine, pyridoxal, pyridoxamine (**B_6**) (Vitamin B_6 is the term applied to a family of 3 related pyridine derivatives),
6. Biotin (Vitamin H), **B_7** or Coenzyme **R,**
7. Folic acid/folate (pteryol glutamic acid) **B_9**, and
8. Cobalamin or cyanocobalamin **(B_{12})**

Q.6. Name vitamin like substances/nutrients/metabolites

Ans. (i) α-Lipoic acid (thioctic acid),
(ii) Para aminobenzoic acid (PABA),
(iii) Choline,
(iv) Inositol,
(v) Carnitine,
(vi) Coenzyme Q (CoQ), and
(vii) Bioflavonoids (**vitamin P**)

Q.7. Name the vitamins that are components of the electron transport chain (ETC).

Ans. (i) Niacin,
(ii) Riboflavin, and
(iii) Ubiquinone.

Q.8. Name the vitamins which are partly synthesized in the intestinal tract by the intestinal flora.

Ans. (i) Vitamin K,
(ii) Thiamine (B_1),
(iii) Riboflavin (B_2),
(iv) Niacin (B_3), and
(v) Pyridoxine (B_6)

Q.9. What do you mean by the term avitaminosis and polyavitaminosis?

Ans. The condition induced by the absence of a single vitamin from the diet is called **avitaminosis** e.g. **avitaminosis** B_1. If the deficiency is multiple, then the term **polyavitaminosis is applied.**

Q.10. What are provitamins?

Ans. Provitamins are substances which as such do not possess any vitamin activity but on conversion give rise to vitamins. For instance provitamins of vitamin A are α, β and γ carotenes.

VITAMIN-A

Q.11. In which tissues carotenes get converted into vitamin-A in our body?

Ans. In the wall of small intestine.

Q.12. Name the plant pigments which are converted into vitamin-A.

Ans. i) α, β, and γ carotenes, and
ii) Cryptoxanthine

Q.13. What happens to the colour of skin in case of carotinaemia?

Ans. Yellow pigmentation.

Q.14. In which conditions carotenes level in blood gets elevated?

Ans. i) Myxoedema,
ii) Diabetes mellitus, and
iii) Chronic nephritis.

Q.15. In which conditions carotenes level in blood gets decreased?

Ans. i) Steatorrhoea, and
ii) Malabsorption syndrome

Q.16. What is the normal level of vitamin 'A' in blood?

Ans. i) 19 - 48 μg/dl (U.K.)
ii) 33 - 63 μg/dl (U.S.)
iii) 30 - 90 μg/dl (Scandinavia)

Q.17. Name the vitamin which does not occur in vegetables, but its precursors remain present in them.

Ans. Vitamin A.

Q.18. What is the biochemistry of beta-carotene?

Ans. Beta-carotene, a provitamin A, belongs to the class of carotenoid pigments. It is a powerful antioxidant. It not only inactivates free radicals but also ensures that the chains of reactions do not proceed in the presence of oxygen.

Q.19. How many molecules of vitamin-A are formed from (i) α-carotene, (ii) β-carotene, (iii) γ-carotene?

Ans. (i) 1 molecule,

(ii) 2 molecules, and
(iii) 1 molecule.

Q.20. Name the structurally related compounds that are commonly referred to as vitamin-A.

Ans. (i) Retinol (Vitamin A alcohol),
(ii) Retinol (Vitamin A aldehyde),
(iii) Retinoic acid (Vitamin A acid), and
(iv) β–Carotene (provitamin A)

Q.21. What are the sources of vitamin-A?

Ans. (i) **Animal sources :** Fish oils, butter, milk, eggs, etc. (this vitamin is found only in animal sources)
(ii) **Indirect sources :** It remains present in **plant tissues** in the form of precursors (**carotenes**), e.g. **carrot,** papaya, mango, yellow leafy vegetables, tomato, yellow corn, etc.
(iii) **Rich and best source in the form of precursor is : carrot (contains carotenes)**.

Q.22. What is the daily requirement of Vitamin-A in various categories?

Ans.

Adults (males)	: 3000 IU (900 mcg)
Adults (females)	: 2300 IU (700 mcg)
Pregnancy	: 2600 IU (770 mcg)
Lactation	: 4300 IU (1300 mcg)

Q.23. How many molecules of vitamin 'A' (retinal) are formed from one molecule of β-carotene?

Ans. Two

Q.24. Name the indirect good plant sources of vitamin-A.

Ans. **Carrots, papaya, mango,** tomato and yellow leafy vegetables (**carrot** is the best source, available throughout the year).

Q.25. Is there any other name of vitamin-A?

Ans. Yes, antiophthalmic or antixerophthalmic vitamin.

Q.26. In which organs vitamin A is stored in the human body?

Ans. Liver, kidneys and to some extent lungs. It's always stored in the ester form.

Q.27. What are the main functions of different vitamin-A compounds?

Ans. (i) **Retinol : in steroid hormone, growth and differentiation,**
(ii) **Retinal :** in visual cycle,
(iii) **Retinoic acid :** in **steroid hormone, growth and differentiation,**
(iv) **β–carotene :** as **an antioxidant,**
(v) **Retinal phosphate :** in the synthesis of glycoprotein.

Q.28. Name the precursors (provitamins) of vitamin A.
Ans. Carotenes.

Q.29. Name the rings which remain present in the structure of β-carotene.
Ans. β-ionone.

Q.30. What does vitamin A deficiency cause?
Ans.
1. **Nyctalopia** (Nightblindness i.e., unable to see in night).
2. **Bitot's spots** (shiny pearly spots of triangular shape occurring on the conjunctiva, are the build-up of **keratin)**.
3. **Xerophthalmia** (conjunctiva & cornea get dried first of all, if not treated in time, then it also damages cornea resulting into blindness.
4. **Xerosis** (cornea gets dried & becomes wrinkled, its shining is lost, if untreated, later on ulcers develop).
5. **Keratomalacia** (ulceration takes place, if untreated, then ulcers damage cornea).
6. **Degeneration** of germinal epithelium occurs, thus affects **reproduction**.
7. **Growth failure** in youngs as the collagenous tissue is affected.

Q.31. Who won Nobel Prize in vision chemistry?
Ans. Professor Wald (1967)

Q.32. Who discovered Vitamin 'A'?
Ans. McCollum

Q.33. What are the biochemical functions of vitamin 'A'?
Ans. (a) **Required for the formation of rhodopsin** (essential for normal vision) i.e., visual function,

(b) **For the formation of glycoproteins,**
(c) **In the regulation of gene transcription,**
(d) Promotion of **gluconeogenesis,**
(e) **Proper healing & maintenance of epithelium,**
(f) Involved in **electron transport chain & oxidative phosphorylation,**
(g) **Proper growth of bones & teeth,** and
(h) Required for the **synthesis of mucopolysaccharides.**

Q.34. What about the concentration of vitamin A activity in β-carotene?

Ans. It has the highest vitamin A activity as upon hydrolysis, it yields two molecules of vitamin A as shown below:

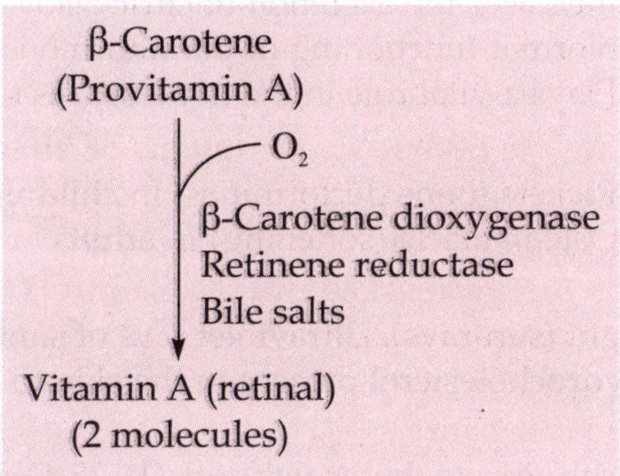

Q.35. What is the normal level of vitamin A in serum?

Ans. 15-50 µg/dl or 0.5 - 2 µmol/L

VITAMIN D

Q.36. What are the active forms of vitamin D?

Ans. (i) 25-hydroxycholecalciferol (25-HCC)
(ii) 1, 25-dihydroxycholecalciferol (1, 25-DHCC).

Q.37. Name the organs which synthesize active forms of vitamin D.

Ans. (i) Formation of 25-HCC takes place in liver.
(ii) Formation of 1, 25-DHCC takes place in the kidneys.

Q.38. Name the precursors of vitamin D.

Ans. (i) **Ergosterol:** It gives rise to ergocalciferol (Vitamin D_2).
(ii) **7-Dehydrocholesterol:** It gives rise to cholecalciferol (vitamin D_3).

Q.39. What is the daily requirement of vitamin D?

Ans. The new 2010 RDA is :
(a) **1-70 years** (including pregnancy & lactation): **600 IU**
(b) **71 years and above : 800 IU**

Q.40. What are the functions of vitamin D?

Ans. (i) Mineralization of bones.
(ii) Absorption of calcium and phosphorus from the intestines.
(iii) Increases the excretion of citric acid.
(iv) Normal functioning of parathormone.
(v) Plays a vital role in the homeostasis of Ca and P.

Q.41. What are the deficiency symptoms of vitamin D?

Ans. (i) Rickets (bone derformities) in children
(ii) Osteomalacia (softening) in adults.

Q.42. What is the cheapest source of vitamin D?

Ans. Sun light (sun-rays). Ultraviolet rays of sunlight convert 7-dehydrocholesterol present in the skin to vitamin D_3.

Q.43. What is calcitriol?

Ans. 1, 25 dihydroxycholecalciferol (1, 25 DHCC) is also known as calcitriol because it contains 3 hydroxyl groups (at 1, 3 and 25 carbons).

Q.44. What is the active form of vitamin D known as?

Ans. 1, 25 DHCC (Calcitriol)

Q.45. How the level of calcitriol regulated in blood?

Ans. Hormonal level of calcitriol in blood is regulated by the feedback control (feedback regulation), its rate of synthesis is modulated by serum levels of Ca, P, PTH and calcitriol itself. The major site of regulation is the enzymic activity **of enzyme α-hydroxylase of kidneys.**

Hypercalcemia decreases the synthesis of calcitriol whereas low dietary intake of calcium and **hypocalcemia** increase it.

Q.46. What is vitamin D_1?

Ans. There is no Vitamin D_1.

Q.47. What is vitamin D_2?

Ans. It is ergocalciferol, a synthetic derivative of plant sterol. It is of importance for humans.

Q.48. What is vitamin D_3?

Ans. It is cholecalciferol, a derivative of cholesterol. Vitamin D_3 is of importance for humans.

Q.49. Is vitamin D_3 active form?

Ans. No

Q.50. What is vitamin D_4?

Ans. It is activated 22-dehydroergosterol, it has got no antirachitic activity, hence of no use for us.

Q.51. What is vitamin D_5?

Ans. It is activated 7-dehydrositosterol, it has got no antirachitic activity, hence of no use for us.

Q.52. What are the various types of rickets?

Ans.
(a) **Renal rickets** (caused due to poor or no synthesis of calcitriol in kidney diseases, such cases respond well to the administration of calcitriol).
(b) **Vitamin D resistant rickets** (in this type, renal tubular reabsorption of phosphate, bicarbonate, glucose and amino acids gets affected).
(c) **Hypophosphatemic rickets** (caused due to defective renal tubular reabsorption of phosphate; they are cured by giving such patients vitamin D along with phosphate preparation).

Q.53. What are the causes of Vitamin D deficiency?

Ans.
(a) Dietary deficiency,
(b) Insufficient exposure to sunlight,
(c) Chronic obstructive jaundice,
(d) Gastrointestinal disorders, and
(e) Prolonged treatment with **anticonvulsant, i.e., antiepileptic drugs, like phenytoin** and certain **antitubercular drugs, like rifampicin.**

Q.54. Besides sunrays (sunlight), what are the other sources of vitamin D.

Ans. **Good sources** : Fish liver oils, margarine (imitation butter) and eggs.
Poor sources : Milk, grains, vegetables and butter.

Q.55. What is hypervitaminosis D?

Ans. Consumption of extremely large doses of vitamin D (500-1,000 times more than the normal requirement) causes **hypervitaminosis D**, the salient features of which are:
(a) Anorexia (loss of appetite),
(b) Increased urinary excretion of Ca & P which may lead to kidney stones (**urinary lithiasis**), and
(c) Renal damage

Q.56. What is William syndrome?

Ans. It is characterized by:
(a) Over dosage of vitamin D,
(b) Hyperparathyroidism,
(c) Infants with hypercalcemia, hypervitaminosis D, aortic stenosis and mental retardation (congenital).

Q.57. Name the provitamins of vitamin D?

Ans. (i) Ergocalciferol (plant source)
(ii) Cholecalciferol (animal source)

Q.58. Where the two hydroxylations take place in 1, 25 dihydroxycholecalciferol?

Ans. (i) Introduction of hydroxyl group at position 25 takes place in the liver.
(ii) Introduction of hydroxyl group at position 1 takes place in the kidneys. Hydroxylation in the kidneys is promoted by parathyroid hormone.

Q.59. What is the name of calcium binding protein of the bone?

Ans. Osteocalcin.

Q.60. How rickets and osteomalacia are corrected?

Ans. They are corrected by giving vitamin D_3.

Q.61. What are the salient functions of vitamin D?

Ans. Recent researches on the mechanism of action of vitamin D have revealed an interesting fact that vitamin D functions more as a hormone than a vitamin for the following reasons :

(i) Vitamin D can be synthesized by the body.
(ii) Vitamin D proper is inactive and is only a storage form, for activity it has to be converted either to 25 hydroxy or 1, 25 dihydroxy compounds.
(iii) It has definite target organs like bone, kidneys, and small intestines (property of hormones).
(iv) The formation of active form of vitamin D_3 is subject to feed back control (property of hormones).
(v) The active form of vitamin D_3 maintains calcium homeostasis along with two other hormones, namely the parathyroid hormone and the calcitonin hormone.
(vi) 1, 25 dihydroxy D_3 resembles steroid hormones in its mode of action. In the intestines, it enters the cell and gets bound to a cytoplasmic receptor molecule. This complex is translocated to the nucleus. It effects an increase in the intestinal absorption of calcium by increasing the synthesis of calcium binding protein.

VITAMIN E

Q.62. What is the other name of vitamin E?

Ans. Tocopherol.

Q.63. How many isomers of tocopherol are known today?

Ans.
(i) α-tocopherol (alfa) (ii) β-tocopherol (beta)
(iii) γ-tocopherol (gamma) (iv) ζ_1-tocopherol ($zeta_1$)
(v) ζ_2-tocopherol ($zeta_2$) (vi) η-tocopherol (eta)
(vii) δ-tocopherol (delta) (viii) ε-tocopherol (epsilon)

Q.64. What are the functions of vitamin E?

Ans. A. **As an antioxidant i.e.:**
(i) Prevents the auto-oxidation of vitamin A and carotenes.
(ii) Prevents the formation of fatty acid peroxidases in the tissues due to the auto-oxidation of unsaturated fatty acids with oxygen.
(iii) Protects lipids of biological membranes against oxygen by acting as an antioxidant.

B. **Prevents rancidity.**

Q.65. What is the daily requirement of Vitamin E?

Ans. (a) **Adults** and **Pregnancy** 15 mg, and
(b) **Lactation** 20 mg or even more upto 1 g

Q.66. What is the source of vitamin E?

Ans. Wheat germ oil & vegetable oils.

Q.67. Which disease is caused due to the deficiency of vitamin E?

Ans. So far, no particular deficiency disease has been reported in human beings, however, **sterility** has been reported in rats.

Q.68. What is the biochemistry of vitamin E?

Ans. Vitamin E (Tocopherol) is a major lipid soluble chain breaking antioxidant which prevents lipid peroxidation in biological membranes as well as lipoproteins.

Q.69. What are the beneficial effects of high intake of vitamin E?

Ans. It's believed that high intake of vitamin E (200-300 mg per day):
(i) Protects against the development of heart diseases.
(ii) Slows down the ageing process.
(iii) Reduces the risk of cancers.

VITAMIN-K

Q.70. What is the daily requirement of vitamin-K?

Ans. Since it is effectively synthesized by the intestinal flora, therefore, its requirement via diet is almost negligible–120-180 mcg.

Q.71. What are the functions of vitamin-K?

Ans. It is required for the coagulation of blood i.e.
(i) It stimulates the production of prothrombin.
(ii) It is also involved in the manufacture or preservation of other blood-clotting factors, including proconvertin, Christmas factor and Stuart factor.

Q.72. Name the diseases caused due to the deficiency of vitamin-K.

Ans. (i) Haemorrhage conditions (excessive bleeding)
(ii) Prolongation in clotting time.

Q.73. What are the chemical names of vitamin-K_1, K_2 & K_3?

Ans. (a) 2- methyl - 3 phytyl-1,4 - naphthoquinone, popularly known as **phylloquinone,**
(b) **Menaquinone**, and
(c) **Menadione**, respectively

Q.74. What are the sources of vitamin-K?

Ans. Green leafy vegetables, soyabean oil, liver etc.

Q.75. What are the main sources of vitamin-K?

Ans. Alfa-alfa (green leafy vegetable), spinach, cabbage, cauliflower, soyabean, whole wheat, liver, pork, etc.

(B_1) THIAMINE

Q.76. What is the daily requirement of vitamin thiamine?

Ans. (a) **Adults** : 1.2 mg, (b) **Pregnancy** : + 0.2 mg
(c) **Lactation** : + 0.3 mg

Q.77. Which disease is caused due to the deficiency of vitamin thiamine?

Ans. **Beriberi** which is manifested by anorexia, weight loss, fatigue & GIT disturbances.

Q.78. Name the biological active form of vitamin B_1.

Ans. Thiamine pyrophosphate (TPP).

Q.79. Is there any other name of TPP?

Ans. Cocarboxylase.

Q.80. What are the biochemical functions of vitamin B_1?

Ans. Thiamine pyrophosphate (TPP) participates as a coenzyme:

(i) In the oxidative decarboxylation of α-keto acids:
 (a) Pyruvic acid → Acetyl CoA
 (b) α-Ketoglutaric acid → Succinyl CoA.

(ii) In the transketolation reaction of hexose monophosphate shunt pathway.

$$\text{D-xylulose-5-PO}_4 + \text{D-ribose-5-PO}_4$$
$$\downarrow$$
$$\text{D-sedoheptulose-7-PO}_4 + \text{D-glyceraldehyde-3-PO}_4$$

Q.81. What are the sources of vitamin B_1?

Ans. Dry peas, beans, soyabeans, bran, rice polishings, legumes, wheat flour, eggs, pork etc.

Q.82. In the deficiency of vitamin thiamine (B_1) which compound gets excreted in increased amount in the urine?

Ans. Pyruvic acid

Q.83. Which compound is formed when thiamine is phosphorylated?

Ans. **Thiamine pyrophosphate,** i.e, TPP (cocarboxylase).

Q.84. In which conditions (diseases), blood pyruvic acid level gets increased?

Ans. i) Diabetes mellitus,
ii) Congestive heart failure,
iii) Diarrhoea,
iv) Digestive disturbances,
v) Severe liver damage, and
vi) Some acute infections.

Q.85. Name the compound formed by the oxidation of thiamine.

Ans. Thiochrome

(B_2) RIBOFLAVIN

Q.86. What is the daily requirement of riboflavin (B_2)?

Ans. (a) Adults : 1.5 mg
(b) Pregnancy : + 0.2 mg
(c) Lactation : + 0.3 mg

Q.87. Why is vitamin B_2 called lactoflavin?

Ans. Since it was first of all isolated from milk, hence called lactoflavin.

Q.88. What are the coenzyme forms of vitamin B_2?

Ans. (i) Flavin mononucleotide (FMN), and
(ii) Flavin adenine dinucleotide (FAD).

Q.89. What are the deficiency symptoms of vitamin B_2?

Ans. Cheilosis, glossitis, seborrheic dermatitis etc.

Q.90. What are the sources of vitamin B_2?

Ans. Germinating seeds, yeast, few intestinal flora, liver, kidney, eggs, cheese, milk, etc.

NIACIN (B_3)

Q.91. Which disease is caused due to the deficiency of vitamin niacin?

Ans. Pellagra = [pelle (skin) + agra (rough)].

Q.92. What are the coenzyme forms of vitamin niacin?

Ans. NAD (Co I) & NADP (Co II)

Q.93. What are the symptoms of Pellagra?

Ans. They mainly include dermatitis of face, neck, knees and breast etc.

Q.94. What are the sources of niacin?

Ans. Liver, kidney, peanuts, dried legumes, milk, egg, fruits, etc.

Q.95. What are the 3 D's symptoms of niacin deficiency?

Ans. (i) Diarrhoea, (ii) Dermatitis, and
(iii) Dementia (headache, depression and forgetfullness).

Q.96. What is the daily requirement of niacin?

Ans. (a) Adults : 20 mg
(b) Pregnancy : + 2 mg
(c) Lactation : + 4 mg

Q.97. Name the vitamin which has got lipid lowering effect.

Ans. Niacin.

Q.98. What are the important functions of NAD & NADP?

Ans. They are required for a number of important oxidation processes.

Q.99. What do you know about the chemistry of niacin (B_3)?

Ans. It is a pyridine derivative and structurally it is pyridine 3-carboxylic acid. The amide form of niacin is known as niacinamide or nicotinamide.

PANTOTHENIC ACID (B_5)

Q.100. What are the sources of pantothenic acid (B_5)?

Ans. Yeast, liver, kidney, egg-yolk, fish, nuts, skimmed milk, molasses, sweet potato, wheat, barley, etc.

Q.101. What is the daily requirement of pantothenic acid?

Ans. Adults : 10 mg

Q.102. What are the deficiency symptoms of vitamin pantothenic acid?

Ans. They may include:

(i) Gastrointestinal symptoms,
(ii) Easy fatigue,
(iii) Changed sleeping pattern,
(iv) Staggering gait,
(v) Mental symptoms, and
(vi) Irritations and **burning sensations of feet.**

burning feet syndrome

Q.103. What are the biochemical functions of pantothenic acid?

Ans. (i) It is a part of coenzyme A which acts as a coenzyme for acyltransferases in acylation and transacylation reactions.

(ii) It helps in the synthesis of some mucopolysaccharides like hyaluronic acid and chondroitin sulphates.

(iii) It helps in the synthesis of gangliosides, blood group polysaccharides, etc.

(iv) It helps in the β-oxidation of fatty acids.

(v) It also helps in the biosynthesis of cholesterol.

Q.104. Which vitamin remains present in the structure of coenzyme A?

Ans. Pantothenic acid.

PYRIDOXINE (B_6)

Q.105. What is the daily requirement of pyridoxine?

Ans. **Adults** : 2 mg, **pregnancy & lactation** : + 2.5 mg

Q.106. Name the three vitamin B_6 (pyridine) derivatives.

Ans. In fact, vitamin B_6 is the term applied to a family of three related pyridine derivatives, i.e.;.

(i) Pyridoxine **(alcohol)**,
(ii) Pyridoxal **(aldehyde)**, and
(iii) Pyridoxamine

Q.107. Name the biologically active form of vitamin B_6?

Ans. Pyridoxal phosphate (PLP)

Q.108. What are the biochemical functions of pyridoxine (B_6)?

Ans. (i) **In transamination reactions.**

(ii) **In decarboxylation reactions,** i.e.,

(a) Histidine ⟶ Histamine

(b) Tyrosine ⟶ Tyramine

(c) Glutamic acid ⟶ γ-aminobutyric acid (GABA)

(iii) **In dehydrases reactions;** i.e.,

(a) Serine ⟶ Pyruvic acid

(b) Threonine ⟶ α-keto butyric acid

(iv) **In transsulphurase reaction:**

Homocysteine ⟶ Serine

(v) **In desulphuration reactions:**

Cystine ⟶ Pyruvic acid

Homocysteine ⟶ α-keto butyric acid

(vi) **In tryptophan metabolism:**

Kynurenine ⟶ Anthranilic acid

(vii) **In the transport of amino acids and in the absorption of amino acids also.**

(viii) In the **synthesis of essential fatty acids (EFA).**

Q.109. What are the deficiency symptoms of vitamin pyridoxine?

Ans. Lesions in the skin.

Q.110. In the deficiency of vitamin pyridoxine (B_6), which compound gets excreted in larger amount in the urine?

Ans. Xanthurenic acid

Q.111. What is the biochemical basis of anaemia due to pyridoxine deficiency?

Ans. Active form of pyridoxine (B_6) is pyridoxal phosphate which acts as a coenzyme for :

(i) Transaminases, (ii) Decarboxylases,

(iii) Dehydrogenases, and

(iv) Also involved in amino acids metabolism.

Heme synthesis starts from succinyl CoA and glycine. ALA synthase requires PP and Mg^{++} as coenzymes. During the synthesis of heme, glycine combines with

ALA synthase - B_6 complex to form **Schiff's base.** Later on, it condenses with succinyl CoA to form α-amino-β-ketoadipic acid and aminolevulinic acid. Pyridoxal phosphate is regenerated. Since it is the most important step in heme synthesis, therefore, deficiency of vitamin B_6 results in anaemia.

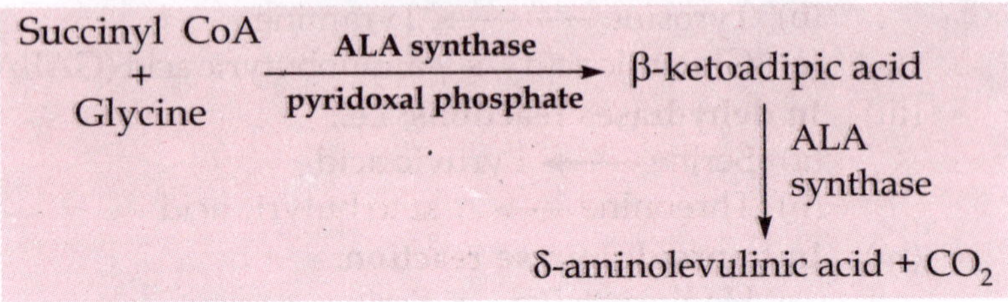

Q.112. What happens in infants due to the deficiency of pyridoxine (B_6)?

Ans. It can lead to convulsions due to a deficiency in γ-aminobutyric acid (GABA), the formation of which from glutamic acid requires pyridoxine as coenzyme

Q.113. Which enzymes require pyridoxal phosphate (PP) as coenzyme?

Ans. Transaminases, etc.

Q.114. Name the drug which induces vitamin B_6 deficiency?

Ans. **Isoniazid (isonicotinic acid hydrazide i.e. INH)** is a drug frequently used for the treatment of tuberculosis. It combines with pyridoxal pyrophosphate to form inactive hydrazone derivatives which inhibit pyridoxal pyrophosphate dependent enzymes. **Another drug penicillamine** also inactivates pyridoxal phosphate dependent enzymes. **Therefore, administration of isoniazid or penicillamine causes vitamin B_6 deficiency.**

BIOTIN (B_7)

Q.115. What is the other name of vitamin biotin?

Ans. Vitamin H.

Q.116. What is the daily requirement of biotin?

Ans. 35- 60 µg (mcg)

Q.117. What are the sources of vitamin biotin?

Ans. Yeast, liver, egg-yolk, kidney, dry legumes, molasses, peanuts, chocolate, tomatoes and milk, etc.

Q.118. What are the main biochemical functions of vitamin biotin?

Ans. It is required as a coenzyme/prosthetic group in CO_2 fixation reactions which are:

(i) Pyruvate $\xrightarrow{\text{carboxylation}}$ Oxaloacetate

(ii) Propionyl CoA $\xrightarrow{\text{carboxylation}}$ Methyl malonyl CoA

(iii) Acetyl CoA $\xrightarrow{\text{carboxylation}}$ Malonyl CoA

(iv) Synthesis of fatty acids

(v) Synthesis of purines and pyrimidines

(vi) Formation of carbamoyl phosphate in the **"urea cycle"**.

Q.119. What are CO_2 fixing or carboxylation reactions?

Ans. Carboxylation reactions are those in which a molecule of CO_2 is added to produce a carboxyl group.

Q.120. Name the antagonists of biotin.

Ans. (i) Desthiobiotin, and

(ii) Biotin sulfonic acid.

FOLIC ACID (B_9)

Q.121. What is the coenzymic form (active form) of folic acid?

Ans. Tetrahydrofolic acid (THF or FH_4).

Q.122. What are the deficiency symptoms of folic acid vitamin?

Ans. (a) **Macrocytic anaemia** with **megaloblastic changes** in the bone marrow,

(b) Diarrhoea & GI disturbances,

(c) Deficiency may block **conversion of homocysteine to methionine,**

(d) Deficiency impairs **DNA synthesis,** and

(e) Deficiency may lead to **neural tube defects in the Ist trimester during pregnancy.**

Q.123. What is the daily requirement of folic acid?

Ans. (a) Adults : 400 μg

(b) Pregnancy : 800 μg

(c) Lactation : 600 μg

(d) Children : 100-300 μg

Q.124. What are the functions of folic acid?

Ans. As a carrier of one carbon moiety.

Q.125. Name one carbon moieties.

Ans. (i) Methyl group ($-CH_3$)

(ii) Formyl group ($-CHO$)

(iii) Hydroxy methyl group ($-CH_2OH$)

(iv) Formimino group ($-CH = NH$).

Q.126. What are the components of vitamin folic acid?

Ans. (a) Pteridine nucleus, (b) PABA, and (c) glutamic acid.

Q.127. Name the antagonists of folic acid.

Ans. (a) **Aminopterin and Amethopterin (methotrexate)**. Both are used as **anticancer drugs** especially in cases of leukemias and choriocarcinomas.

(b) **Pyrimethamine (anti-malarial drug)**

(c) **Sulfonamides & Trimethoprim (anti-bacterial drugs)**

Q.128. Name the reactions mediated by one carbon moiety.

Ans. (i) Glycine ⟶ serine

(ii) Ribonucleotides ⟶ deoxyribonucleotides

(iii) Ethanolamine ⟶ choline

(iv) Uracil ⟶ thymine

(v) Guanidoacetic acid ⟶ creatine

(vi) Norepinephrine ⟶ epinephrine

(vii) In purine synthesis (i.e. C-2 and C-8 positions in purine skeleton come from one carbon moiety).

Q.129. Name the sources of folic acid.

Ans. **Fresh** green leafy vegetables, **fresh** fruits, cereals, pulses, eggs, etc.

Q.130. What happens to the excretion of FIGLU in urine in whom there is found deficiency of vitamin folic acid?

Ans. When there is a deficiency of folic acid, there is a lack of tetrahydrofolic acid, so that, FIGLU is not removed by the reaction as shown above; rather it accumulates in the blood **and then excreted in urine in increased amount.**

Sometime, however, in cases of folic acid deficiency such an increase is not found because there is insufficient histidine. For this reason, histidine loading was introduced and urine FIGLU determined after such a load. This has increased the sensitivity of the test considerably.

Q.131. Whether way folic acid is involved in the metabolism of histidine, if yes, then how?

Ans. Histidine is converted to *N*-formiminoglutamic acid (FIGLU) which then reacts with tetrahydrofolic acid to give glutamic acid and N^5-formiminotetrahydrofolic acid, a reaction catalyzed by the enzyme FIGLU transferase as shown below:

Histidine

↓

Urocanic acid

↓

Imidazole-propionic acid

↓

N-Formiminoglutamic acid

\+

Folic acid ⟶ Tetrahydrofolic acid

↓

Glutamic acid + N^5-formiminotetrahydrofolic acid

Q.132. In the deficiency of vitamin folic acid, which compound gets excreted in increased amount in the urine?

Ans. Formiminoglutamic acid.

COBALAMIN (VITAMIN B_{12})

Q.133. Name the coenzymes (coenzymic forms) of vitamin B_{12}.

Ans. (a) Methylcobalamin, (b) Adenosylcobalamin, (c) Hydroxycobalamin, (d) Aquocobalamin, (e) Nitrocobalamin, and (f) Cyanocobalamin.

Q.134. What are the main functions of methylcobalamin?

Ans. (i) It is required for the health of nervous system, i.e., prevents degeneration of nervous tissue. Indications of a potential deficiency of B_{12} in humans include **numbness** and **tingling of fingers or toes,** later on **inability of gait** and **paralysis.**

(ii) It's required for the conversion of **homocysteine** to **methionine** which acts as a **methyl donor** for a large number of reactions that need a **methyl** group, including the **synthesis of myelin, serotonin, dopamine, noradrenaline, DNA** and **phospholipids.**

Q.135. In the deficiency of vitamin B_{12}, which compound gets excreted in increased amount in the urine?

Ans. Methylmalonic acid **(it's a marker of B_{12} deficiency).**

Q.136. What are the main functions of adenosylmethionine?

Ans. (i) It's a coenzyme for the conversion of L-methylmalonyl-CoA into succinyl CoA which feeds into TCA cycle.

(ii) It's also used by the enzyme **leucine aminomutase** to convert β-leucine into L-leucine and vice-versa.

Q.137. What is the modus operandi of the synthesis of vitamin cobalamin (B_{12})?

Ans. Vitamin B_{12} is synthesized by microbes that occur in the rumen (the first stomach chamber) of the cows and sheep. From the rumen, it is transferred to the muscle and other tissues, which other animals and human eat.

Q.138. What are the good dietary sources of vitamin B_{12}?

Ans. (i) **Good sources :** Liver, kidney, meat, and fish

(ii) **Fair sources :** Eggs, fermented foods, milk, cheese, curd, etc

Q.139. What does severe deficiency of vitamin B_{12} cause?

Ans. Its severe deficiency may lead to degeneration of certain motor and sensory tracts of spinal cord; if the degeneration continues for sometime, treatment with vitamin B_{12} may not correct it. **Initial numbness and tingling of fingers or toes may, without treatment, progress to inability of gait and paralysis afterwards.**

Q.140. What are the advantages of taking high amount of vitamin B_{12} in elderly people?

Ans. High vitamin B_{12} level in elderly people may protect them against the atrophy of brain or shrinkage associated with **Alzheimer's disease and impaired cognitive (sensation) functions.**

Q.141. Which test is meant for the detection of pernicious anemia?

Ans. Schilling test

Q.142. Which vitamin is used in Schilling test?

Ans. Vitamin B_{12}.

Q.143. What is the daily requirement of vitamin B_{12}?

Ans. (a) Adults : 1 - 2 µg (b) Pregnancy : 2 - 6 µg

(c) Lactation : 2 - 8 µg (d) Children : 0.2 - 1 µg

Q.144. What are the other names of vitamin B_{12}?

Ans. Cobalamin and cyanocobalamin.

Q.145. What does the deficiency of vitamin B_{12} cause?

Ans. **Pernicious anaemia.**

Q.146. Why is vitamin B_{12} called as cyanocobalamin?

Ans. Because it contains:

(i) Cyano group, and

(ii) Cobalt atom in its structure.

Q.147. Name the vitamin in which cobalt remains present as a prosthetic group entity.

Ans. Vitamin B_{12}

VITAMIN-C (Ascorbic acid)

Q.148. What does the deficiency of ascorbic acid (vitamin-C) cause?

Ans. Scurvy resulting in anaemia, pain in joints, haemorrhages from the mucous membranes of the G.I. tract, swelling & bleeding of gums.

Q.149. What is the daily requirement of vitamin-C?

Ans. (a) Adults : 45 mg, (b) Pregnancy : 60 mg
(c) Lactation : 80 mg

Q.150. What are the sources of vitamin-C (ascorbic acid)?

Ans. (i) **Citrus fruits like** amla, lemon, guava, orange, pineapple etc.
(ii) **Vegetables like** cauliflower, tomatoes, spinach, green pepper, potatoes etc.

Q.151. What are the biochemical functions of vitamin-C?

Ans. (i) In the synthesis of collagen.
(ii) In the synthesis of carnitine in the liver.
(iii) In tissue respiration.
(iv) Necessary for the absorption of iron by reducing ferric form to ferrous form.
(v) In the synthesis of steroidal hormones both in the adrenal cortex and the corpus luteum.
(vi) As cofactor in the following reactions :
(a) *p*-Hydroxyphenylpyruvic acid

$$\downarrow$$

Homogentisic acid
(involved in phenylalanine metabolism in the conversion as shown above)
(b) Folic acid → Folinic acid
(c) Dopamine → Norepinephrine

Q.152. Name the versatile vitamin.

Ans. **Vitamin C** has been considered as a versatile vitamin taking into account its vast clinical importance.

Q.153. What is the rich animal source of vitamin-C?

Ans. **Adrenal cortex**

Q.154. What is the normal level of vitamin-C in blood?

Ans. 0.7-1.2 mg%.

Q.155. Are human beings capable of synthesizing vitamin-C in the body?

Ans. No, because of the absence of enzyme L-gulonooxidase.

Q.156. In the deficiency of vitamin-C, which compound gets excreted in increased amount in the urine?

Ans. Homogentisic acid

Q.157. What is the biochemistry of vitamin-C?

Ans. Vitamin C (ascorbic acid) is known as a **first line antioxidant and a powerful inhibitor of lipid peroxidation.**

Q.158. Milk is found to be poor in which vitamins & minerals.

Ans. Vitamin C, vitamin D, B_1 and Iron

Q.159. How does vitamin-C participate in collagen synthesis?

Ans. It acts as a coenzyme and brings about post-translational modification while protocollagen is converted to collagen. Ascorbic acid is needed for the conversion of proline and lysine (present in protocollagen) to hydroxyproline and hydroxylysine respectively.

MISCELLANEOUS

Q.160. What is another name of coenzyme 'Q'?

Ans Ubiquinone

Q.161. What is the role of ubiquinone?

Ans. In electron transport chain.

Q.162. Another name of bioflavonoids is :

Ans. Vitamin P.

Q.163 What is the normal level of blood lactic acid?

Ans. 6 to 18 mg/dl

Q.164 In which disorder, blood lactic acid level gets increased?

Ans. Liver disorders, because liver converts lactic acid to glycogen.

Q.165. In which disorder, level of blood lactic acid gets decreased?

Ans. Hypoxia.

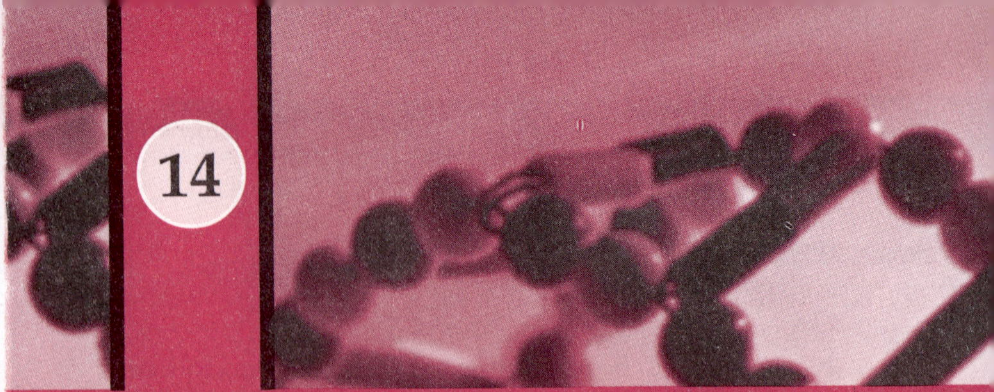

14

NUTRITION, MILK AND ENERGY REQUIREMENT

Q.1. Why do we require food?

Ans. We require food for energy purposes. When food gets burnt in the animal system - it liberates energy. This energy energises the cells for their proper functioning.

Q.2. What are the components of food?

Ans.
(i) Carbohydrates
(ii) Lipids
(iii) Proteins
(iv) Minerals
(v) Vitamins, and
(vi) Water

Q.3. What is the definition of a 'Calorie'?

Ans. A 'Calorie' is defined as the amount of heat required to raise the temperature of 1 kg of water by one degree centigrade.

Q.4. How is caloric value of food estimated?

Ans. It is estimated by burning the food in a closed metal chamber (bomb calorimeter), filled with oxygen and placed in a known mass of water.

Q.5. What is a balanced diet?

Ans. A balanced diet is one which contains all the constituents of food in proper proportion so as to provide energy and nutritional requirements for proper growth and reproduction.

Q.6. What is the latest unit of measuring energy?

Ans. Joules.

Q.7. What is the average calorie requirement of human beings of different categories?

Ans.
(i) Sedentary : 2500 Cal
(ii) Light work : 3000 Cal
(iii) Moderate work : 3500 Cal
(iv) Heavy work : 4000 Cal and above as per the physical exertion done.

Q.8. How much calories does one obtain by burning 1 g of carbohydrate, 1 g of protein and 1 g of lipid in the human body?

Ans.
1 g carbohydrate = 4 Cal
1 g protein = 4 Cal
1 g lipid = 9 Cal

Q.9. What is the unit of measuring energy?

Ans. Kilocalorie or Calorie (large calorie).

Q.10. What is respiratory quotient (RQ)?

Ans. $$RQ = \frac{\text{Volume of } CO_2 \text{ produced}}{\text{Volume of } O_2 \text{ consumed}}$$

Q.11. What is the RQ for carbohydrates' oxidation?

Ans. It is 1.

Q.12. What is Basal Metabolic Rate (BMR)?

Ans. It is the amount of energy required just to maintain the basic physiologic functions when a person is at complete rest. BMR is proportionate to lean body weight and to surface area. It is higher in males than females.

Q.13. Which conditions should be borne in mind before measuring BMR of a person?

Ans.
(i) Subject should be at rest.
(ii) Subject should be awaken.
(iii) Subject should be in a warm environment (temperature 20—25°C).
(iv) Measurement should be done at least 12 hours after the last meal.

Q.14. In which conditions/diseases BMR is found to be raised?

Ans. Fever and hyperthyroidism.

Q.15. In which states/diseases, BMR is found to be low?

Ans. Hypothyroidism and starvation.

Q.16. What is Specific Dynamic Action (SDA)?

Ans. It is defined as the extra heat production over and above the caloric value of a given amount of food when used by the body.

Example: An amount of protein which contains 100 Kcal (25 g) when metabolized in the body, the heat production is not 100 Kcal but 130 Kcal. This extra 30 Kcal is the product of the SDA of protein. Similarly, in the body, a 100 Kcal portion of carbohydrate produces 105 Kcal. This extra heat is due to the activity of tissues metabolizing these foodstuffs.

Q.17. Which has got highest SDA among carbohydrates, lipids and proteins?

Ans. Proteins. The SDA of proteins is 30%.

Q.18. What is the protein sparing action of carbohydrates and lipids?

Ans. Carbohydrates and lipids make themselves available for energy purposes, and thus, spare proteins are still important purposes like body building/building of tissues etc.

Q.19. What are the food sources of lipids?

Ans. Butter, cheese, vegetable oils and their hydrogenated products, nuts, eggs, soyabeans, ice creams, some fatty meats, oily fishes, pulses, etc.

Q.20. Name essential fatty acids (EFA).

Ans. (i) Linoleic acid,
(ii) Linolenic acid, and
(iii) Arachidonic acid.

Q.21. Name some polyunsaturated fatty acids (PUFA).

Ans. (i) Linoleic acid,
(ii) Linolenic acid, and
(iii) Arachidonic acid.

Q.22. What do you understand by 'Biological value of protein'?

Ans. This is defined as the per cent of the absorbed protein nitrogen which is retained in the body and not excreted in the urine. A high biological value, therefore, indicates a high degree of utilization of the amino acids of the protein.

Q.23. Do animal proteins have high biological value than the vegetable proteins?

Ans. Yes, animal proteins like liver, meat, egg and milk have high biological value than the vegetable proteins like those of cereals, pulses and vegetables.

Q.24. What are the biological values of egg (whole), egg (white), cow's milk, fish, pork and liver?

Ans. 94%, 83%, 85%, 70-80%, 77% and 77% respectively.

Q.25. What are the biological values of ragi, rice, bengal gram, red gram (arhar dal), cashew nut, barley and black gram?

Ans. 89%, 86%, 76%, 74%, 72%, 71% and 64% respectively.

Q.26. What is the daily requirement of protein for adults?

Ans. 0.9 g/kg body weight or say, roughly 1 g/kg body weight.

Q.27. What is the extra daily requirement of proteins in case of pregnancy and lactation?

Ans. 10 and 20 g respectively

Q.28. What is the daily requirement of proteins in case of infants and children?

Ans. 1.5-2.0 g/kg body weight.

Q.29. What are the signs and symptoms of low protein diet?

Ans. (i) Anemia,

(ii) Hypoalbuminemia,

(iii) Edema, and

(iv) Peptic ulcer.

Q.30. What are the signs and symptoms of diet low in protein and choline?

Ans. (i) Fatty liver, and

(ii) Cirrhosis.

Q.31. What is Kwashiorkor?

Ans. It has its highest incidence between the age group of 1-4 years and is caused due to **poor intake of proteins** in the diet. The syndrome is characterized by :

(i) Growth failure
(ii) Retarded development
(iii) Loss of appetite
(iv) Mental apathy
(v) Hypoalbuminemia leading to edema
(vi) Diarrhoea
(vii) Pellagrous skin lesions
(viii) Dermatosis, etc.

Q.32. What is marasmus?

Ans. It is still aggravated form of Kwashiorkor where the diet besides being **deficient in proteins** is also **markedly deficient in calories.** The syndrome is characterized by :

(i) Subnormal body weight
(ii) Severe wasting of muscles and loss of subcutaneous fat
(iii) Atrophy and wasting of muscles lead to thinning of limbs and abdominal wall as a result of which ribs become prominent
(iv) Hepatic cirrhosis
(v) Gastrointestinal disturbances
(vi) Skin becomes thin, dry, shrunken, wrinkled and almost devoid of subcutaneous fat

Q.33. What is the literal meaning of marasmus?

Ans. Neglected child.

Q.34. What should be the extra daily requirement of calories during pregnancy?

Ans. By about 300-400 calories.

Q.35. What should be the extra daily requirement of calories during lactation?

Ans. By about 500-700 calories.

Q.36. What are the food sources of first class proteins?

Ans. Meat, fish, eggs, wheat, milk etc.

Q.37. What do you understand by the term first class proteins?

Ans. First class proteins are those which do contain all essential amino acids (EAA) - which are **eight** in number and possess **good digestibility** and **easy absorbability.**

Q.38. Which is the most respected complete biological protein?

Ans. **Casein of milk** has been respected as a complete biological protein primarily due to the presence of all the essential amino acids and secondarily due to its very good digestibility and absorbability.

Q.39. What are the food sources of second class proteins?

Ans. (i) Various dry legumes (pulses),
(ii) Peas,
(iii) Beans,
(iv) Corns, etc.

Q.40. Name sulfur containing amino acids.

Ans. (i) Cystine,
(ii) Cysteine,
(iii) Methionine,
(iv) Homocysteine,
(v) Selenocysteine, and
(vi) Selenomethionine

Q.41. Name selenium containing amino acids.

Ans. (i) Selenocysteine, and
(ii) Selenomethionine.

Q.42. Name some first class proteins and their sources.

Ans. (i) Lactalbumin of milk,
(ii) Casein of milk,
(iii) Ovalbumin of egg,
(iv) Glutenin of wheat,
(v) Globulin of cottonseed, and
(vi) Edestin of hempseed.

Q.43. Name some second class proteins and their sources.

Ans. (i) Legumelin of soyabean,
(ii) Gliadin of wheat ,
(iii) Zein of corn,
(iv) Hordein of barley, and
(v) Legumin of pea.

Q.44. What is the number of essential amino acids?

Ans. Eight.

Q.45. Is there any formula to remember essential amino acids?

Ans. MTTVILPLy

Q.46. Name the essential amino acids.

Ans. (i) Methionine,
(ii) Threonine,
(iii) Tryptophan,
(iv) Valine,
(v) Isoleucine,
(vi) Leucine,
(vii) Phenylalanine, and
(viii) Lysine.

Q.47. Is there any amino acid which is considered to be essential for infants?

Ans. Histidine.

Q.48. How much amount of proteins is secreted daily in the milk of a lactating woman?

Ans. 10-20 g.

Q.49. Name the proteins found in egg-white.

Ans. Ovalbumin and ovoglobulin (**both of very high biological value**).

Q.50. Name the protein found in egg-yolk.

Ans. Ovovitellin (**of very high biological value**).

Q.51. Does raw egg-white contain any other protein? If yes, what is its action?

Ans. It contains a thermolabile basic protein called **avidin, which reduces the absorption of vitamin biotin.**

Q.52. What is the effect of cooking of eggs?

Ans. It is beneficial because it :
(i) Inactivates both avidin and the antidigestive factor.
(ii) Slows the rate of the absorption of cholesterol, thus hypercholesterolaemia is checked.
(iii) Kills the bacteria, thus egg borne infections like salmonella do not infect the man, otherwise the infection of salmonella is very bad.

Q.53. In which portion of egg remains present cholesterol?

Ans. Yolk

Q.54. Which minerals are found in abundance in eggs?

Ans. (i) Calcium,

(ii) Phosphorus, and

(iii) Iron.

Q.55. What is the caloric value of an average egg?

Ans. About 165 calories.

Q.56. Name the proteins found in milk.

Ans. (i) Lactalbumin,

(ii) Lactaglobulin, and

(iii) Casein.

Q.57. Name the phosphoprotein found in milk.

Ans. Casein.

Q.58. What is the effect of boiling the milk on the digestibility of casein?

Ans. It gets increased.

Q.59. Which vitamins are poor in milk?

Ans. Vitamins C, K and D.

Q.60. Is milk poor in iron?

Ans. Yes.

Q.61. What are the calorie values of cow's, buffaloes and human milk per 100 ml?

Ans. 69, 109 and 67 calories.

Q.62. What is the calorie value of butter?

Ans. 720 cal/100 g.

Q.63. Is butter very rich in vitamin A and carotenes?

Ans. Yes.

Q.64. What is the calorie value of desi ghee?

Ans. 830-890 calories/100 g.

Q.65. What is the colostrum?

Ans. It's viscous, yellow liquid secreted from the mammary glands during the first 4-5 days after parturition (child birth).

It is richer than mature milk in:
(i) Proteins,
(ii) Vitamin A,
(iii) Vitamin D,
(iv) Vitamin B complex group,
(v) Tocopherols, and
(vi) Calcium.

and poorer than mature milk in:
(i) Casein,
(ii) Fat, and
(iii) Lactose.

Q.66. Are eggs rich in cholesterol?
Ans. Yes.

Q.67. Name the enzymes that act on various lipids.
Ans. (i) Lipases,
(ii) Lecithinases (phospholipases) i.e. lecithinase A, B, C and D,
(iii) LCAT (lecithin cholesterol acyl transferase),
(iv) Sphingomyelinase,
(v) Hexosaminidase A and B,
(vi) Gm_1-β-galactosidase, etc.

Q.68. How much cholesterol remains present in 100 g of hen egg yolk and whole egg?
Ans. 1500 and 550 mgs respectively.

Q.69. What is the effect of polyunsaturated fatty acids on the level of blood cholesterol?
Ans. They lower it.

Q.70. Name some saturated fatty acids.
Ans. (i) Palmitic acid,
(ii) Caproic acid,
(iii) Caprylic acid,
(iv) Stearic acid,
(v) Lauric acid, and
(vi) Myristic acid, etc.

Q.71. Where does fat digestion mainly take place?
Ans. Intestine.

Q.72. Name some unsaturated fatty acids.

Ans.
(i) Oleic acid
(ii) Palmitoleic acid } monounsaturated
(iii) Erucic acid
(iv) Linoleic acid (diunsaturated)
(v) Linolenic acid (triunsaturated)
(vi) Arachidonic acid. (quadraunsaturated)

Q.73. Would you give preference to vegetable oils over animal oils or fats in your diet?

Ans. Vegetable oils as they possess PUFA which have a tendency to lower blood cholesterol level.

Q.74. What is the daily requirement of lipids for a normal person?

Ans. 80 gm.

Q.75. What is the normal level of cholesterol in serum?

Ans. 150-200 mg/dl (more to say, now it's 150-180 mg%)

Q.76. What is the normal level of HDL cholesterol in serum?

Ans.
(i) 30-63 mg% (men)
(ii) 35-75 mg% (women)

Q.77. What is the normal level of LDL cholesterol in serum?

Ans. 40-130 mg%.

Q.78. What is the normal level of serum triglycerides?

Ans. 30-140 mg/dl.

Q.79. What is atherosclerosis?

Ans.
(i) It is a disease of the hardening of the arteries.
(ii) It is a disease primarily concerned with the intimal layer of the artery.
(iii) It is characterized by the thickening and loss of elasticity of the arterial walls by the excessive deposits of cholesterol and other lipids.
(iv) It occurs in the aorta, coronary, cerebral, renal, iliac and femoral arteries.

Q.80. Which enzymes are used to disintegrate thrombus (clots) in the cardiac arteries and elsewhere?

Ans.
(i) **Streptokinase** (from streptococcus strain),
(ii) **Tissue plasminogen activator (TPA)**, which, in turn, converts blood protein plasminogen into

plasmin which has got the capability to dissolve blood clots.

(iii) **Urokinase** (from urine),

(iv) **Nattokinase** (from fermented soyabean)

(v) **Bromelain** (an enzyme extracted from pineapple),

(vi) **Serrapeptase** (enzyme isolated from silk worm).

Q.81. How does enzyme streptokinase act (mechanism)?

Ans. **Streptokinase** is an extracellular protein, extracted from certain strains of beta hemolytic streptococcus. It is a non-protease plasminogen activator that activates **plasminogen to plasmin,** the enzyme that degrades fibrin clot through its specific lysine binding site; it is used, therefore, as a drug in **thrombolytic therapy.**

Q.82. What are the main functions of lipids in the body?

Ans. (i) They play an important role in the diet by helping in the absorption of fat soluble vitamins i.e. A, D, E and K.

(ii) Lecithins prevent development of fatty livers.

(iii) Nutritional cirrhosis of liver is caused in the deficiency of dietary choline which is a part of lecithin molecule.

(iv) They serve as the more important source of energy in the diet of hard workers such as wrestlers, athletes, etc.

Q.83. What are the side effects of excess intake of fats (lipids)?

Ans. Excess fat intake should be avoided because it causes:

(i) An increase in the adiposity,

(ii) Hypercholesterolaemia,

(iii) Ketosis, etc. which all are undesirable, and

(iv) High fat consumption is also associated with the cancer of the breast and the colon.

Q.84. What are the sources of essential fatty acids?

Ans. (i) Linseed oil,

(ii) Cottonseed oil,

(iii) Peanut oil,

(iv) Corn oil,

(v) Soyabean oil,

(vi) Egg-yolk,
(vii) Rapeseed oil,
(viii) Fish viscera, etc.

Q.85. What are the main functions of essential fatty acids?

Ans. **To serve as precursors of** :

(i) Leukotrienes,
(ii) Prostaglandins,
(iii) Thromboxanes,
} act as 'local hormones'

(iv) **Important constituents of lipoproteins,**

(v) Disposal and Oxidation of cholesterol requires EFAs, thus **reduce level of cholesterol in blood,** and

(vi) The phospholipids of cell membranes and mitochondrial membranes contain EFA. In EFA deficiency, the changes in the integrity of these membranes affect many metabolic processes. Red cell membranes become fragile and may get easily hydrolyzed.

Q.86. What are the main sources of saturated fatty acids in the diet of human beings?

Ans. (i) Meat of ruminants,
(ii) Dairy products, and
(iii) Hard margarine.

Q.87. What are the important risk factors of atherosclerosis?

Ans. (i) High blood pressure,
(ii) Diabetes mellitus,
(iii) High blood cholesterol,
(iv) Smoking, and
(v) Obesity

Q.88. What is the percentage of the contribution of carbohydrates in the total calories furnished by the diet by a normal man daily?

Ans. 40-80%.

Q.89. What is the minimum requirement of carbohydrates per day by a normal man?

Ans. At least 100 g of carbohydrates are required per day by a normal healthy adult in order to avoid ketosis, excessive protein catabolism and other undesirable responses.

Q.90. What is the normal requirement of carbohydrates per day by a normal healthy adult?

Ans. Nearly 400 g.

Q.91. What is the food value of eating raw potato?

Ans. Potato consists of starch granules surrounded by an envelope of cellulose. If a raw potato is eaten or even if it is chewed thoroughly, it will pass through the digestive tract as such without yielding any calories and appear undigested in the feces. **A raw potato has, therefore, got no food value.**

Q.92. What is the food value of a cooked potato?

Ans. If the potato is heated, then the cellulose envelope bursts and the content is then available for digestion and production of calories. This is an example of a food which has got no food value in the raw state but has **a very high food value in the cooked state.**

One medium size boiled potato gives nearly 83 calories.

Q.93. Cellulose forms an integral part of the fibrous part of vegetables and fruits. Is the consumption of cellulose in the diet by human beings useful or not?

Ans. Although, cellulose is not digested by human beings because of the absence of corresponding enzyme i.e. cellulase in our system but side-by-side its consumption is very useful because it provides **roughage** to the fecal matter and thus helps preventing **colon cancers.** Contrarily, **'Cellulase'** is found in abundance in ruminants (cattles) whose main food is grasses which contain mainly cellulose.

Q.94. What do you mean by fibre rich diet?

Ans. A rich (high) fibre diet means which is rich in:

(i) Cellulose, (ii) Hemicellulose,
(iii) Lignin, (iv) Gums,
(v) Pectins, and
(vi) Pentosans

Q.95. What is the advantage of taking high fibre diet?

Ans. In humans, a high fibre diet exerts beneficial effects **by causing water retention** during passage of food along the gut **and thereby producing larger, softer feces.**

A high fibre diet has also been found to be associated with reduced incidence of:

(i) Constipation,
(ii) Diverticulosis,
(iii) Appendicitis,
(iv) Cancer of the colon,
(v) Cardiovascular diseases,
(vi) Diabetes mellitus (reduces the absorption of glucose by the intestines),
(vii) Hypercholesterolaemia (by binding the bile salts and setting them apart, as a result of which, the concentration of bile salts reaching the liver by entero-hepatic circulation gets decreased, and
(viii) Heart diseases.

Q.96. What is the RQ for fat oxidation?

Ans. About 0.7

Q.97. What is the RQ for protein oxidation?

Ans. About 0.8

Q.98. What is the level of Hb in blood below which one is said to be anaemic?

Ans. 10 g%

Q.99. What are the main causes of nutritional anaemia?

Ans. Less intake of iron, folic acid and vitamin B_{12}.

Q.100. What is the energy requirement of women of the age group of 18-65 years per day?

Ans. Nearly 2200 kcal/day.

Q.101. What is the daily energy requirement of a pregnant woman?

Ans. + 300 i.e., nearly 2500 kcal/day.

Q.102. What is the calorific requirement of boys (15-18 yrs) per day?

Ans. 2800 kcal/day

Q.103. What is the calorific requirement of girls (15-18 yrs) per day?

Ans. 2300 kcal/day

Q.104. What are the good edible sources of fibre?

Ans. Rice bran, wheat bran, legumes, fruits, vegetables and leafy greens.

Q.105. What is the action of invertase upon sucrose in the small intestine?

Ans. It gets hydrolyzed to its constituent units, i.e., glucose and fructose.

Q.106. Strictly speaking which is the main EFA out of the three, i.e., linoleic, linolenic and arachidonic acids.

Ans. **Linoleic acid,** which can not be synthesized whereas other types of EFA can be synthesized, provided there is linoleic acid.

Q.107. What is the percentage of proteins in egg?

Ans. 12.5%

Q.108. Which vitamins are found in eggs?

Ans. It contains B_2 and some other members of B group as well as vitamins A and D.

Q.109. Name the antagonist of biotin which is found in raw eggs. What is the effect of cooking / boiling of eggs upon that antagonist?

Ans. Avidin which gets destroyed upon cooking/boiling.

Q.110. Which important minerals are found to be missing in milk?

Ans. Fe and Cu

Q.111. Name the fatty acids found in milk.

Ans. Butyric, caproic, caprylic, capric, lauric, myristic, palmitic, stearic and oleic acids with very little amount of PUFA.

Q.112. What do you understand by the term "requirement of hemopoietic factors"?

Ans. By the above term, we mean the intake of:

(i) Iron,
(ii) Folic acid, and
(iii) Vitamin B_{12}

Q.113. What are the various biochemical parameters for the clinical diagnosis of nutritional anaemias?

Ans. Biochemical parameters include assessment of the following in blood :

(i) Iron,
(ii) Ferritin and transferrin receptor,
(iii) Folic acid, and
(iv) Vitamin B_{12} status, etc.

Q.114. By which technique, serum ferritin and serum transferrin receptors are determined?

Ans. ELISA

Q.115. Which vegetable is supposed to prevent enlargement of prostate and what is that chemical?

Ans. Tomato; lycopene

Q.116. Which mineral is found in abundance in banana and what beneficiary effect it has got on heart?

Ans. Potassium; **strengthens artery walls** of the heart.

Q.117. Why intake of limited amount of chocolates is good for heart?

Ans. Their limited intake is good for keeping heart healthy as chocolates contain compounds known as **'flavonoids'** which have a tendency to prevent the formation of blood clots. Besides, flavonoids are also responsible for proper blood circulation in the arteries as a result of which there is least risk of heart attacks.

Chocolates are also responsible to increase the capacity of **'antioxidants'** which help preventing the formation of such **elements which otherwise may cause cancers in human beings.** Flavonoids come in the mixture of chocolates from **'coke'** of which they are made-up of, but all chocolates do not possess the same quantity of flavonoids as it depends upon the technique of the preparation of chocolates. **Some techniques destroy flavonoids partially or fully.**

Chocolates should be eaten with care but not in excess as their excess consumption is side-by-side responsible for increasing fat (adiposity) in the body.

Q.118. What are the major constituents of milk?

Ans (i) Carbohydrates (Lactose)
(ii) Fats, and

(iii) Proteins, i.e.,
 (a) Caseinogen **(a phosphoprotein)**,
 (b) Lactalbumin, and
 (c) Trace of lactoglobulin

Q.119. Which minerals and vitamins are found in good amount in milk?

Ans. (i) Calcium,
(ii) Phosphorus,
(iii) Vitamin A, and
(iv) B_2 (Riboflavin)

Q.120. What is the significance of the determination of milk phosphatase activity?

Ans. This is carried out to check the reliability of pasteurization. If this has been done efficiently, the milk should show no phosphatase activity.

Q.121. What is the composition of humans and cow's milk?

Ans. It is as mentioned below:

	Human's (Range %)	**Cow's (Range %)**
Water	82—90	82—90
Protein	1—2	2.5—4.5
Caseinogen	0.8 (average)	2.85 (average)
Albumin	0.5 (average)	0.55 (average)
Fats	2.0 —4.5	2.5—5.5
Lactose	0.1—0.4	0.6—0.9
Calcium	0.018—0.042	0.09—0.17
Phosphorus	0.010—0.020	0.07—0.12

Q.122. Is the consumption of desi ghee in moderate amount is good for health, if yes then why?

Ans: Consumption of animal fat i.e; desi ghee in moderate amount is good for health because of the following good properties, namely:

(i) It contains 40 percent good fat which has a tendency to reduce bad cholesterol in the body.

(ii) Has some antioxidants which prevent degenerative changes and certain bad conditions including ageing.

That is why, it's consumed since ages. However, it should be consumed in excess taking into account the physical activity one performs daily.

Q.123. What is coprophagy?

Ans: Some animals like rats, deers, have a tendency to eat their own faeces, this phenomenon is called as **'Coprophagy'.**

Q.124. Name the types of nutritional anemias.

Ans. There are three types, namely :

(a) Iron deficiency anemia,

(b) Nutritional megaloblastic anemia, and

(c) Anemia of protein-caloric malnutrition (PCM)

Q.125. What is the daily loss of iron in menstruating females and pregnant females?

Ans. 0.6 mg and 1.5 mg respectively.

Q.126. What is the main cause of lathyrism?

Ans. Consumption of **'Khesari dal',** the grain of which resembles that of Arhar/Toor/ Tuvar dal (Cajanus cajan).

Q.127. What is the name of toxin which remains present in *'Khesari dal'* responsible for lathyrism?

Ans. β-oxalyl amino alanine (BOAA).

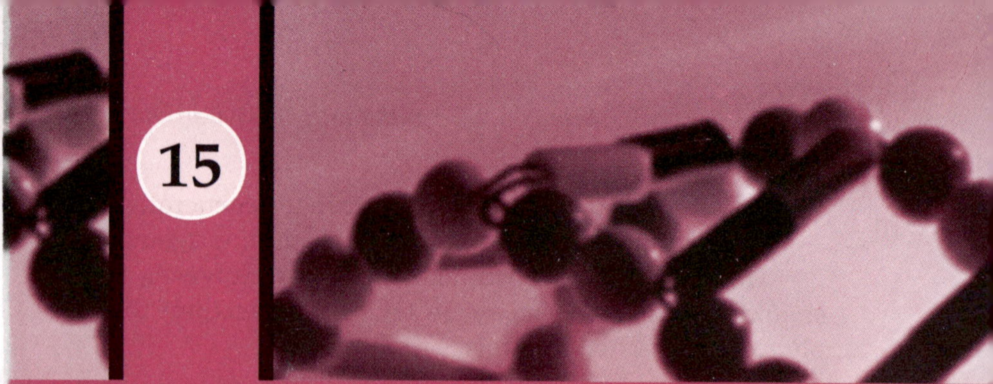

15 Bile and Liver Function Tests

Q.1. From where bile is secreted?

Ans. By the polygonal cells of the liver.

Q.2. Where bile is stored in the human body?

Ans. Gall bladder.

Q.3. How much amount of bile is secreted per day?

Ans. 500-1000 ml

Q.4. What is the colour of the bile and what are its functions?

Ans. It's colour is golden yellow and it has several metabolic functions in the body:

(i) Bile acids have got the property to lower the surface tension, promote lipid emulsification and thereby increase the surface area exposed to the enzyme lipase.

(ii) Bile salts help in the absorption of fat soluble vitamins i.e., A, D, E and K.

(iii) Bile acids are also required for the gastrointestinal absorption of cholesterol and formation of cholesterol esters.

(iv) Biliary excretion represents the main pathway for the excretion of many substances such as Na^+, K^+, Cl^-, creatinine, glucose, penicillin, cholesterol, bilirubin, etc.

Q.5. How much amount of bile pigments is excreted in human urine per day?

Ans. 1-2 mg.

Q.6. How much amount of bile pigments is excreted in human faeces per day?

Ans. 50-250 mg.

Q.7. What is the composition of bile?

Ans. It consists of:

(i) Water
(ii) Bile acids
(iii) Bile pigments
(iv) Mucin
(v) Lipids (fatty acids, cholesterol, phospholipids, etc.)
(vi) Inorganic substances.

Q.8. What is the capacity of gall bladder?

Ans. 50-60 ml.

Q.9. Which hormone is responsible for the initiation of the construction of gall bladder?

Ans. Cholecystokinin.

Q.10. What is the composition of gall stones?

Ans. They are usually made-up of :

(i) Cholesterol,
(ii) Bile pigments,
(iii) Soaps,
(iv) Calcium phosphate,
(v) Calcium carbonate, and
(vii) Protein material

Q.11. Name the bile acids found in the bile.

Ans. (i) Cholic acid
(ii) Chenodeoxycholic acid
(iii) Deoxycholic acid.

Q.12. How does the synthesis of bile acids take place?

Ans. From cholesterol.

Q.13. Name the bile pigments.

Ans. (i) Bilirubin (yellow)
(ii) Biliverdin (brown)
(iii) Mesobilirubin

(iv) Mesobilirubinogen
(v) Stercobilin
(vi) Stercobilinogen etc.

Q.14. What is the main bile pigment of faeces?

Ans. Stercobilin (brown).

Q.15. Name the main bile pigment of urine.

Ans. Urobilin.

Q.16. What is the normal level of bilirubin in serum?

Ans. 0.2-1.0 mg per cent.

Q.17. What are the main biochemical functions of the liver?

Ans. (i) To form urea.
(ii) To synthesize plasma proteins.
(iii) To form bile acids.
(iv) To detoxify endogenous and foreign compounds.
(v) It is the main site for the metabolism of carbohydrates, lipids and proteins, etc.

Q.18. What are the various liver function tests commonly performed?

Ans. (i) GOT (AST)
(ii) GPT (ALT)
(iii) Serum total proteins, A/G ratio
(iv) Serum alkaline phosphatase
(v) γ-glutamyl transferase
(vi) Serum bilirubin
(vii) Serum cholesterol
(viii) Prothrombin time.

Q.19. What is the importance of liver function tests?

Ans. (i) To assess the severity of liver damage.
(ii) To differentiate different types of jaundice.
(iii) To find out the presence of latent liver disease.

Q.20. What is the normal level of total serum proteins?

Ans. 6.0-8.0 g/dl.

Q.21. What is the normal level of serum albumin?

Ans. 3.5-5.0 g/dl.

Q.22. What is the normal level of serum globulins?

Ans. 2.3-3.6 g/dl.

Q.23. What is the normal level of fibrinogen in plasma?

Ans. 0.3-0.6 g/dl.

Q.24. What is the normal A/G ratio?

Ans. 1.2 to 1.5.

Q.25. In which conditions, total proteins in blood get elevated?

Ans. Multiple myeloma.

Q.26. Name the conditions in which total proteins are low.

Ans.
(i) Neoplastic disease
(ii) Malnutrition
(iii) Kwashiorkor syndrome
(iv) Cirrhosis of liver and other liver disorders.

Q.27. In which condition fibrinogen in blood gets lowered?

Ans. Cirrhosis of liver.

Q.28. In which condition fibrinogen in blood gets raised?

Ans. Infections.

Q.29. Where are proteins synthesized in our body?

Ans. Liver.

Q.30. What happens to A/G ratio if there is liver damage?

Ans. Synthesis of albumin gets decreased, hence A/G ratio gets lowered.

Q.31. How will you separate different proteins from each other?

Ans. By electrophoresis.

Q.32. In case of nephrotic syndrome, what will be the abnormality in the urine sample?

Ans. Urine will exhibit the presence of albumin.

Q.33. Why albumin appears first in the urine?

Ans. Albumin is low molecular weight and smaller in size as compared to globulin and hence gets filtered by the glomeruli first.

Q.34. What are the functions of plasma proteins?

Ans.
(i) They serve as building block units for cellular, subcellular and organic structures.
(ii) They act as defence against infections by way of protein antibodies.

(iii) They help in maintaining osmotic pressure.
(iv) They act as buffers.
(v) They are carriers of various metabolites.

Q.35. In which conditions cholesterol level in blood gets raised?

Ans. (i) Diabetes mellitus
(ii) Hypothyroidism
(iii) Obstructive jaundice
(iv) Cirrhosis of liver
(v) Nephrotic syndrome, etc.

Q.36. In which conditions cholesterol level in blood gets decreased?

Ans. (i) Acute hepatitis
(ii) Malnutrition
(iii) Anaemia
(iv) Occasionally in hyperthyroidism.

Q.37. For what SGOT and SGPT stand?

Ans. SGOT stands for Serum Glutamate Oxaloacetate Transaminase and SGPT stands for Serum Glutamate Pyruvate Transaminase.

Q.38. What is the normal level of serum bilirubin?

Ans. 0.2-1.0 mg/dl.

Q.39. Name the reaction by which bilirubin is estimated colorimetrically.

Ans. Van den Burgh reaction.

Q.40. How is bilirubin formed?

Ans. It is formed as a result of breakdown of hemoglobin.

Q.41. In which diseases/disorders level of bilirubin in blood gets raised?

Ans. (i) Obstructive jaundice
(ii) Hemolytic jaundice
(iii) Neonatal jaundice and
(iv) Hepatitis.

Q.42. What is direct (conjugated) bilirubin?

Ans. Bilirubin diglucuronide is called direct bilirubin. It is water soluble.

Q.43. What is the normal level of direct i.e. conjugated bilirubin?

Ans. 0.0-0.2 mg/dl.

Q.44. What is indirect bilirubin?

Ans. Bilirubin bound to protein (specifically albumin) is called indirect bilirubin. It is water insoluble.

Q.45. What is the normal level of indirect (unconjugated) bilirubin?

Ans. 0.2 to 0.8 mg/dl.

Q.46. In which diseases direct bilirubin gets raised?

Ans. (i) Hepatitis
(ii) Obstructive jaundice.

Q.47. In which diseases indirect bilirubin (unconjugated) gets raised?

Ans. (i) Hemolytic jaundice
(ii) Neonatal jaundice.

Q.48. What is jaundice or icterus?

Ans. This is due to the accumulation of bilirubin in the blood which imparts yellow colouration in the conjunctiva of eyes, mucous membrane and skin after a certain concentration.

It is often, though not always, connected with liver and biliary tract disease.

Q.49. At which concentration in blood jaundice is usually visible?

Ans. When serum bilirubin exceeds 2.4 mg/dl

Q.50. What is the significance of the measurement of bilirubin in serum?

Ans. It gives a measure of the intensity of jaundice. Higher values are found in obstructive jaundice than in hemolytic jaundice.

Q.51. What is obstructive jaundice?

Ans. This is caused due to the blockage or obstruction of the hepatic or common bile duct as a result of which bile pigment is believed to pass from the blood into the liver cells as usual but fails to be excreted.

This obstruction may arise either due to tumor or gallstone or any other cause in the hepatic or common bile duct.

Q.52. When does bilirubin appear in urine?

Ans. In obstructive jaundice.

Q.53. What is hemolytic jaundice?

Ans. This is due to increased rate of breakdown of red blood cells (e.g., pernicious anemia) leading to increased rate of the formation of bile pigments which in fact exceeds the capacity of the liver to remove the pigments.

Q.54. What is the most common cause of unconjugated hyperbilirubinemia?

Ans. It's the transient neonatal "physiological jaundice". This hyperbilirubinemia results from an accelerated hemolysis and an immature hepatic system for the uptake, conjugation and secretion of bilirubin.

Q.55. Name the bile salts.

Ans. (i) Sodium glycocholate

(ii) Sodium taurocholate.

Q.56. Which enzyme is found to be deficient in physiological jaundice?

Ans. UDP - glucuronyl transferase.

Q.57. What is the name of the substrate on which UDP-glucuronyl transferase acts?

Ans. UDP-glucuronic acid.

Q.58. What is hyperbilirubinemic toxic encephalopathy or kernicterus?

Ans. Since the increased bilirubin is unconjugated, it is capable of penetrating the blood-brain barrier when its concentration in plasma exceeds that which can be tightly bound by albumin (20-25 mg/dl). This can result in a hyperbilirubinemic toxic encephalopathy or kernicterus.

Q.59. What is the treatment of infants suffering from kernicterus?

Ans. (i) Phenobarbital therapy

(ii) Exposure to visible light (phototherapy).

Q.60. What is Crigler-Najjar syndrome, Type-I, congenital non-hemolytic jaundice?

Ans. It's a rare autosomal recessive disorder of humans and is caused due to a primary metabolic defect in the conjugation of bilirubin. It is characterized by severe congenital jaundice due to the inherited absence of bilirubin UDP-glucuronyl transferase activity in hepatic tissues. The disease is usually fatal within the first 15 months of life. Phenobarbital therapy has no role in this type of jaundice, however, phototherapy plays some role.

Q.61. What is Crigler-Najjar syndrome, Type-II?

Ans. This rare inherited disorder seems to result from a milder defect in the bilirubin conjugating system and has a more benign course. It has been proposed that the genetic defect may involve the hepatic UDP-glucuronyltransferase that adds the second glucuronyl group to bilirubin monoglucuronide.

Phenobarbital therapy in large doses plays role in this type of jaundice.

Q.62. What is Gilbert's disease? Which enzyme is found to be missing in this disorder?

Ans. (i) It is a state of unconjugated hyperbilirubinemia.
(ii) Enzyme missing is bilirubin UDP-glucuronyl transferase or its activity gets reduced.

Q.63. What is Dubin-Johnson syndrome?

Ans. It's an autosomal recessive disorder which consists of conjugated hyperbilirubinemia in childhood or during adult life, is caused due to defect in the hepatic secretion of conjugated bilirubin into the bile. Characteristically, in such patients, the hepatocytes in the centrilobular area contain an abnormal pigment that has not been identified so far.

Q.64. How many molecules of δ-aminolevulinic acid give rise to porphobilinogen?

Ans. Two.

Q.65. What is hepatitis-E?

Ans. HEV is a icosahedral non-enveloped RNA virus approximately 32-34 nm in diameter. The virus is shed in the faeces of the infected patients and hence spread from person-to-person by the faecal/oral route. Contaminated drinking water has been implicated as the major source in all the epidemics. The virus causes an acute **self-limiting hepatitis.**

Outbreaks occur most commonly after the recession of the flood water during the monsoon. These climatic conditions along with the poor standards of personal hygiene create a scene for epidemics that are usually associated with this infection.

Q.66. How many types of viral hepatitis known today?

Ans. Five i.e., A,B,C,D and E.

Q.67. What are the abbreviations for viral hepatitis A, B, C, D and E?

Ans. HAV IgM, HBs Ag, HCV, HD IgM and HEV IgM.

Q.68. What is alcoholic hepatitis?

Ans. Patients with alcoholic hepatitis exhibit a broad range of clinical features ranging from asymptomatic hepatomegaly and minimal test abnormalities to severe liver injury with progressive jaundice, coagulopathy, fever, leucocytosis, ascites, renal failure, and encephalopathy. The diagnosis is usually made on clinical grounds, supported by serum AST level less than 300 to 500 IU/L and an AST–to–ALT ratio of greater than two.

Measurement of gamma glutamyltransferase (GGT) may also be helpful in diagnosing alcohol abuse.

Q.69. What is the best test for liver function?

Ans. Estimation of serum bilirubin.

Q.70. How much haemoglobin is catabolised each day?

Ans. 7.5 g

Q.71. Which type of viral hepatitis is most common and prevalent these days?

Ans. India has approximately **40 million chronic hepatitis B** carriers. A number of serologic tests are available to establish the diagnosis of HBV infection. Hepatitis B surface antigen (HBsAg) is the first marker detectable is serum, preceding elevations in serum aminotransferases as well as the onset of symptoms.

Q.72. How much bilirubin is produced each day from the catabolism of 7.5 g haemoglobin?

Ans. 250 mg

Q.73. Which substance is formed by the reduction of biliverdin?

Ans. Bilirubin

Q.74. How is bilirubin conjugated and excreted through bile?

Ans. It gets conjugated with two molecules of glucuronate supplied by UPP-glucuronate. This reaction is catalysed by **bilirubin glucuronyl transferase.** Bilirubin diglucuronide is excreted into the bile canaliculi against a concentration gradient by an active energy dependent process.

Q.75. What is jaundice and its types?

Ans. Jaundice is a clinical condition characterized by yellow colour of the white portion of the eyes (sclerae) and skin. It occurs due to increased concentration of bilirubin in blood.

There are mainly 3 types of jaundice.

(a) Hemolytic jaundice : It is associated with increased hemolysis of RBCs.

(b) Hepatic jaundice : It is due to the defect/impairment in the functioning of liver.

(c) Obstructive jaundice : It is caused by an obstruction in the bile duct that prevents the passage of bile into the intestine.

Q.76. What do you know about the jaundice due to genetic defects?

Ans. There are certain hereditary disorders that cause jaundice e.g., Crigler-Najjar syndrome type-I and type-II (enzyme defect UDP-glucuronyl transferase).

Q.77 Which type of groups does the structure of bilirubin contain?

Ans. Pyrrole groups.

Q.78 How many pyrrole groups are there in the structure of bilirubin?

Ans. Four

Q.79 How biliverdin is formed from bilirubin?

Ans. It is formed by mild oxidation of bilirubin wherein two hydrogen atoms are removed from the central methane ($-CH_2-$) bridge of bilirubin so that biliverdin has three methyne ($-CH=$) links.

Q. 80. What is the colour of biliverdin?

Ans. Dark green

Q. 81 What are the chief constituents of gastric juice?

Ans.
a) HCl, secreted by the parietal cells
b) Pepsinogen, secreted by the chief cells
c) Rennin, which converts caseinogen to casein.
d) The haemopoietic factor, absence of which is responsible for the development of pernicious anaemia, and
e) Mucus.

Q.82 From which substance bilirubin is formed and in which tissues are formed?

Ans. It is formed from haemoglobin in the reticulo-endothelial system (spleen, bone marrow, Kupffer cells in the liver).

Q.83. Which responses are responsible for the secretion of gastric secretion?

Ans.
a) Psychic factors, sight, taste, smell, and even in extreme circumstances, the thought of food which all are mediated by the vagus nerve.
b) Gastrin a hormone secreted by the gastric mucosa when food is present in the stomach.
c) The presence of some products of digestion in the intestine.

Q.84. Of which substances pancreatic calculi are made-up of?

Ans.
i) Calcium carbonate,
ii) Calcium phosphate,
iii) Traces of magnesium salts, and
iv) Small amounts of protein and fats.

Q.85. What is AIDS Cholangiopathy?

Ans. Acquired immuno deficiency syndrome (AIDS) cholangiopathies are infectious and caused by organisms that were not known previously to infect the biliary tree. **Cryptosporidium** is the most common organism. The clinical presentation usually includes abdominal pain, diarrhoea and cholestatic liver diseases manifested by threefold to tenfold elevations in serum ALP and mild elevations in aminotransferase enzymes. Jaundice is uncommon.

Q.86. Name the rate limiting enzyme of bile acid synthesis.

Ans. 7-α-hydroxylase

Q.87. What is the medicinal use of chenodeoxycholic acid?

Ans. It's used as a drug to dissolve gallstones. Surgery is required when stones obstruct the bile duct, or to remove the inflammed gallbladder.

Q.88. How cholesterol esters are hydrolyzed to free cholesterol and fatty acids?

Ans. By a lysosomal enzyme called **acid lipase** within the cells.

Q.89. What does deficiency of acid lipase cause?

Ans. A genetic deficiency of this enzyme causes accumulation of cholesterol esters and TAG in tissues; the condition is known as **Wolman's disease.**

Detoxification/Detoxication/Biotransformations/Metabolism of Xenobiotics

Q.1. What is detoxification?

Ans. It is a biochemical change occurring in the body whereby foreign molecules that are toxic in nature are converted to comparatively harmless compounds which are more readily excretable.

Q.2. What is the main site of detoxication?

Ans. Liver.

Q.3. Where are large number of detoxifying enzymes located in the cells?

Ans. On the endoplasmic reticulum.

Q.4. What are the various processes (mechanisms) of detoxication?

Ans. (i) Oxidation, (ii) Reduction, (iii) Hydrolysis, and (iv) Conjugation

Q.5. Give the examples of detoxications.

Ans. **Oxidation:**

(i) Benzene ⟶ Phenol
(ii) Benzyl alcohol ⟶ Benzoic acid
(iii) Meprobamate ⟶ Hydroxymeprobamate

Reduction:

(i) Picric acid ⟶ Picramic acid
(ii) *p*-Nitrobenzene ⟶ *p*-Nitrophenol

Hydrolysis:

(i) Atropine ⟶ Tropic acid

(ii) Acetylsalicylic acid (aspirin) ⟶ Salicylic acid

Conjugation :

(i) Benzoic acid $\xrightarrow[\text{acid}]{\text{glucuronic}}$ Benzoyl glucuronide

(ii) Benzoic acid $\xrightarrow{\text{glycine}}$ Hippuric acid

(iii) Indole $\xrightarrow{H_2SO_4}$ Indoxyl sulphate

(iv) *p*-Aminobenzoic acid

↓ acetic acid

p-Acetylaminobenzoic acid

Q.6. Which is the main biochemical disposal process of normal or foreign components out of various processes of detoxication?

Ans. Oxidation.

Q.7. Which compound is formed when choline fraction of phospholipids gets hydrolyzed by bacterial action in the large intestine?

Ans. Neurine.

Q.8. Is neurine a toxic substance or not?

Ans. Yes, it is a toxic substance of low order.

Q.9. Which compounds are formed when amino acids are decarboxylated by the action of intestinal bacteria?

Ans. Ptomaines.

Q.10. Whether the 'Ptomaines' are toxic substances or not?

Ans. Yes, they are toxic amines.

Q.11. Which enzyme brings about the detoxication of cyanides?

Ans. Rhodanase (Rhodanese)

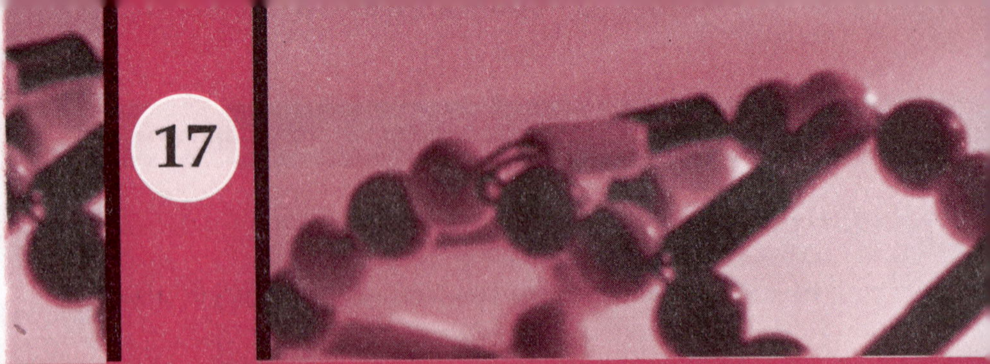

17

HORMONES

Q.1. What are hormones?

Ans. Hormones are the chemical substances that act like messenger molecules in the body. After being secreted in one part of the body, they travel to other parts of the body through blood stream where they help control functioning of cells and organs.

For example, insulin is a hormone that is secreted by the β-cells of the pancreas; when it's released in the blood, it helps regulate the level of sugar in the blood.

Q.2. What is the difference between hormones and the enzymes?

Ans.

	Hormones	Enzymes
1.	Their site of origin is generally far from the site of action	1. Enzymes do their work at the site where they are produced
2.	Hormones have to be discharged in the blood before carrying the reaction	2. Enzymes exhibit their action in the cell
3.	Hormones can be either proteins, or small peptides or amino acids or steroids	3. Enzymes are only protein in nature

Q.3. Name second messengers?

Ans. Cyclic-AMP, cGMP, inositol triphosphate (IP_3) and Calcium ions (Ca^{2+}).

Q.4. How cyclic AMP is formed?

Ans. It is formed from ATP by the action of enzyme adenyl cyclase in the presence of magnesium ions.

$$ATP \xrightarrow[Mg^{2+}]{\text{adenyl cyclase}} c\text{-}AMP$$

Q.5. Name the hormones secreted by pancreas.

Ans. (i) Insulin (β-cells),
(ii) Glucagon (α-cells),
(iii) Gastrin and somatostatin (δ-cells), and
(iv) Pancreatic polypeptide (γ-cells)

Q.6. What is the chemical nature of insulin?

Ans. It is a hypoglycaemic hormone meaning by it has a tendency to decrease blood sugar level. It is proteinous in nature.

Q.7. For the first time who discovered the presence of insulin and in which year?

Ans. Banting, Best and Macleod in 1921-22.

Q.8. From where insulin hormone is secreted in our system?

Ans. It is secreted from the β-cells of the islets of Langerhans found in the pancreas.

Q.9. How many types of cells are found in islets of Langerhans? What are their functions?

Ans. It contains three types of cells, viz.:
(i) α-cells (smaller number): which are responsible for the secretion of glucagon.
(ii) β-cells (many in numbers): which are responsible for the secretion of insulin
(iii) δ-cells (few in number): which are responsible for the secretion of gastrin and somatostatin.

Q.10. How much insulin is secreted per day by the human pancreas?

Ans. Nearly 2 mg i.e. 50 units.

Q.11. Who discovered the structure of Insulin and in which year?

Ans. Frederick Sanger in 1951.

Q.12. In which year Sanger was awarded Nobel Prize for finding out complete amino acid sequence of the protein bovine insulin?

Ans. 1958.

Q.13. Was Sanger awarded Nobel Prize for second time also? If yes, in which year and what was his contribution?

Ans. Yes, he was awarded Nobel Prize for the second time in 1980 for his work in determining the base sequence of nucleic acids.

Q.14. What is the molecular weight of human insulin?

Ans. 5,808 daltons; it is a dimer of an α-chain & a β-chain, which are linked together by disulfide bonds.

Q.15. What is the metal which remains present in insulin?

Ans. Zinc.

Q.16. What is the nature of glucagon?

Ans. It is a hyperglycaemic hormone, meaning by it has a tendency to raise blood sugar level.

Q.17. How many amino acids are present in the structure of glucagon?

Ans. A linear peptide of **29** amino acids.

Q.18. Name the principal hormones of the thyroid gland.

Ans. Thyroxine (T_4) and Triiodothyronine (T_3).

Q.19. For what T_3 and T_4 stand?

Ans. T_3 stands for triiodothyronine and T_4 stands for tetraiodothyronine or thyroxine.

Q.20. Which is more active T_3 or T_4?

Ans. T_3 (4-10 times more potent than T_4).

Q.21. What is the cause of goitre?

Ans. Deficiency of hormone thyroxine.

Q.22. From which amino acid the biosynthesis of thyroxine takes place?

Ans. Tyrosine.

Q.23. What is Wolf Chaikoff effect?

Ans. High amount of iodine has been found to inhibit the organification of iodine which is known as Wolf Chaikoff effect.

Q.24. What are the main functions of thyroid hormones?

Ans. (i) BMR: In hyperfunctioning of thyroid gland, BMR increases and vice-versa.

(ii) Intestinal absorption of glucose is increased.

(iii) In males lack of thyroid hormones is likely to cause complete loss of libido (sexual desire); whereas on the other hand much more excess of thyroid hormones causes impotence.

(iv) In females, excess of thyroid hormones causes menorrhoea or polymenorrhoea which means excessive and frequent menstrual bleeding, respectively. Lack of thyroid hormones may cause irregular period or even total amenorrhoea.

Q.25. Name the goitrogenic foods.

Ans. (i) Cauliflower

(ii) Broccoli (a variety of cauliflower with greenish flower head)

(iii) Cabbage.

Q.26. What is the most practicable way of supplying iodine to the humans?

Ans. Through diet in the form of iodized salt (NaI or KI).

Q.27. What are the hormones of parathyroid glands?

Ans (i) Parathormone

(ii) Calcitonin

Q.28. How the secretion of parathormone is regulated?

Ans. Secretion of parathormone is regulated by the concentration of serum calcium. If the blood calcium is low, parathormone secretion gets increased and vice versa.

Q.29. What are the main functions of parathormone (PTH) and calcitonin (Cl)?

Ans. Their main function is to control calcium and phosphate metabolism in a balancing manner.

Q.30. What is the normal level of serum calcium?

Ans. 9-11 mg%

Q.31. What is the normal level of inorganic phosphate in serum?

Ans. (i) 2.5 - 4.8 mg% (adults)
(ii) 4.0 - 7.0 mg% (children).

Q.32. Which hormones are secreted from adrenal medulla?

Ans. (i) Epinephrine (adrenaline)
(ii) Norepinephrine (noradrenaline).

Q.33. What is the difference between epinephrine (adrenaline) and norepinephrine (noradrenaline)?

Ans. (i) Structural difference: Epinephrine is methylated one whereas norepinephrine is a non-methylated form.

(ii) Epinephrine is mainly secreted from adrenal medulla whereas norepinephrine is released mainly at nerve endings.

(iii) Epinephrine is released in blood and then acts at various organ tissues whereas norepinephrine (noradrenaline) acts only at the site of release because of nerve ending.

(iv) Epinephrine increases heart rate whereas norepinephrine decreases it.

(v) Epinephrine is responsible for anxiety, anger etc. because it affects central nervous system whereas norepinephrine has got no effect on CNS.

Q.34. Name the hormones of anterior pituitary.

Ans. (i) TSH (Thyroid stimulating hormone or thyrotropin)
(ii) ACTH (Adrenocorticotropic hormone)
(iii) GH (Growth hormone) or STH (Somatotrophin hormone)
(iv) Prolactin
(v) FSH (Follicle stimulating hormone)
(vi) LH (Luteinizing hormone).

Q.35. Which types of hormones are synthesized from adrenal cortex?

Ans. It synthesizes three classes of hormones, i.e.:
(i) Glucocorticoids
(ii) Mineralocorticoids, and
(iii) Sex hormones.

Q.36. How many hormones are synthesized from adrenal cortex?

Ans. Nearly 50.

Q.37. What is the other name of mineralocorticoid and what is it's function?

Ans. Aldosterone, the main function of which is the maintenance of electrolyte balance.

Q.38. Name the most important member of the glucocorticoids family.

Ans. Hydroxycorticosterone or cortisol (compound 'F').

Q.39. From which substance steroidal hormones are synthesized?

Ans. Acetyl coenzyme A.

Q.40. What is the most important function of glucocorticoids and how does it happen?

Ans. Anti-inflammatory action, possibly by inhibiting proliferation of fibrous connective tissue by fibroblasts.

Q.41. In which diseases cortisone has been considered to be of great value?

Ans. (i) Rheumatoid arthritis (ii) Rheumatic fever
(iii) Asthma (iv) Hay-fever
(v) Inflammatory eye diseases
(vi) Addison's disease, etc

Q.42. Name the male sex hormones.

Ans. Androgens, of which testosterone is the most important one.

Q.43. Name the female sex hormones.

Ans. (i) Estrogen, and
(ii) Progesterone

Q.44. What are the functions of estrogen?

Ans. (i) Responsible for the development of sex organs at puberty.

(ii) Also responsible for the development of secondary sex characteristics like texture and distribution of hair, texture of skin, character of the voice and distribution of body fat.

(iii) To a large extent also responsible for the rebuilding of the uterine endometrium after menstruation.

Q.45. What are the functions of testosterone?

Ans. (i) Stimulates development of male external genitalia in the foetus.

(ii) Responsible for secondary male characteristics like beard, facial and body hair, moustaches, deep voice, etc.

(iii) Responsible for secondary male sex organs like prostate, seminal vesicles, penis, etc.

(iv) Responsible for promoting growth of the body i.e. skeletal size.

(v) Responsible for the growth of seminiferous tubules and spermatogenesis.

(vi) It regulates the secretion of gonadotropins from the anterior pituitary.

Q.46. What are the functions of progesterone?

Ans. (i) The prime function of progesterone is the induction of the progestational changes of the uterine mucosa.

(ii) It also causes an increase in the vascularity and secretory activity of the mucosa, a condition essential for the nidation (implantation) of the fertilized ovum.

(iii) It inhibits uterine motility.

Q.47. Name the hormones of gastrointestinal tract.

Ans. (i) Secretin

(ii) Gastrin

(iii) Cholecystokinin (CCK)

(iv) Gastric-Inhibitory Polypeptide (GIP)

(v) Vasoactive Intestinal Polypeptide (VIP)

(vi) Motilin

(vii) Substance-P.

Q.48. What is Zollinger-Ellison syndrome?

Ans. Hypersecretion of gastrin by gastrin producing tumors of the pancreas or duodenum or hyperplasia of gastrin producing cells in the presence of gastric antrum is responsible for the well known Zollinger-Ellison syndrome.

Q.49. What is Verner-Morrison syndrome?

Ans. It occurs when tumors grow in the pancreas or neural tissue in the abdomen which secrete vasoactive intestinal polypeptide (VIP). Such tumors have bean named as "VIPomas".

The syndrome is characterized by pancreatic cholera in which there is severe watery diarrhoea with alkalosis and hypokalaemia.

Q.50. What are the hormones of posterior pituitary?

Ans (i) Vasopressin (hexapeptide i.e., contains six amino acids in its structure).

(ii) Oxytocin (octapeptide i.e., contains eight amino acids in its structure).

Q.51. What are the functions of vasopressin?

Ans. (i) It is an antidiuretic hormone (ADH) which stimulates the active reabsorption of water by the renal tubules. The absence or deficiency of this hormone causes 'Diabetes insipidus' which is characterized by excessive water excretion.

(ii) It also has slight "presser" activity, that is, it constricts blood vessels and raises the blood pressure.

(iii) It promotes glycogenolysis.

Q.52. What are the functions of oxytocin?

Ans. (i) It stimulates muscular contraction of the uterus during childbirth.

(ii) It stimulates milk ejection from the mammary glands during lactation.

Q.53. Which hormone is secreted by the parathyroid glands?

Ans. Parathormone

Q.54. What is the function of parathyroid glands?

Ans. They regulate the supply, distribution and metabolism of calcium and phosphorus in the body.

Q.55. What is hyperthyroidism?

Ans. It is accompanied by physiologic effects and symptoms that are the opposite of those observed in **hypothyroidism.** One of the most severe condition is **Graves' disease** or **exophthalmic goitre** This disorder is characterized by an enlargement of the entire gland, **the 'goitre'**, an elevated BMR, weight loss, and a typical protrusion of the eyeballs-hence the adjective "exophthalmic". The condition can be relieved by surgical removal of the thyroid gland, administration of radioactive iodine or usage of thyroid-inhibiting drugs. In most cases, a goitre is a tumour or growth of the thyroid gland, and can be treated surgically with much success.

A simple goitre is caused by a dietary deficiency of iodine. The gland enlarges in an attempt to compensate for the lack of iodine. The goitre is practically not injurious to health until it becomes large enough to cause undue pressure upon the trachea and other nearby structures.

Salient features are :

(1) It is a state in which thyroid gland is too active, as a result of which a condition known as exophthalmic goitre occurs.

(2) A common symptom of this disease is the bulging of the eyes.

(3) This disease is also known as **'GRAVES'** or **'BASEDOW'S'** disease.

(4) BMR is high

(5) Nitrogen metabolism gets increased

(6) Hair are fine

(7) Body's temperature remains above the normal

(8) Patient is nervous and irritable

(9) His IQ is above than normal

(10) He or she is underweight

(11) His/her heartbeats are generally faster and irregular.

Q.56. What is Hypothyroidism?

Ans. Hypothyroidism in adults produces a condition called Myxedema, characterized by a low BMR, thickness and puffing of the skin, coarse and brittle hair and fingernails, and a general mental and physical lethargy. Administration of thyroid extract is the treatment of this situation (disease).

In hypothyroidism, the child becomes a dwarf or cretin. A cretin grows slowly (stunted growth) and has a low mentality (low I.Q.), his hair are scanty and coarse and his skin is thick and dry and low BMR.

Q.57. Name the principal hormone of the thyroid gland.

Ans. Thyroxine.

Q.58. By which amino acid thyroxine is synthesized by the thyroid gland?

Ans. Tyrosine.

Q.59. How is thyroxine synthesized?

Ans. By tyrosine and iodine which should remain present in the diet. Food does not contain free iodine but rather iodide, which is converted to iodine by the thyroid gland itself.

Q.60. Where thyroxine is stored and in which form?

Ans. It is stored in the thyroid gland in the form of thyroglobulin, a protein complex in the form of a large colloid.

Q.61. What is the utility of thyroid function tests?

Ans. In a patient with thyroid dysfunction, if TFT are performed, the results would be normally as given below:

(a) Thyronormalcy (euthyroid) : Normal T_3, normal T_4 and normal TSH.

(b) Hypothyroid (underactive thyroid) : Low T_3, low T_4, and elevated TSH.

(c) Hyperthyroid (overactive thyroid) : Elevated T_3, elevated T_4, and suppressed TSH.

Q.62. What is ectopic hormone syndrome, give examples?

Ans. It's a syndrome, in which there is production of hormones by the "wrong tissue" (e.g., production of parathyroid hormone (PTH) and ACTH by malignant cells in the case of lung cancer. These syndromes, generally, involve a rather restricted number of peptide hormones but a large and apparently diverse number of tissues.

Q.63. What is multiple endocrine neoplasia (MEN) syndrome?

Ans. It's a syndrome in which there is a peculiar familial clustering of neoplasia of several endocrine glands. The production of excessive amounts of peptide or catecholamine hormones, often with one tissue making several, is a feature of such type of syndrome.

Q.64. What is the full form of POMC?

Ans. Pro-opiomelanocortin

Q.65. What happens when thyroglobulin molecule is degraded?

Ans. It releases T_4 and T_3 molecules.

Q.66. What is the primary effect of parathyroid hormone?

Ans. (i) Serum calcium elevating action with a concomitant
(ii) Plasma inorganic phosphate decrease

Q.67. What is the action of cathepsin-B upon parathyroid hormone (PTH)?

Ans. It cleaves PTH into two fragments, **PTH_{1-36}** and **PTH_{37-84}**

Q.68. What is the molecular weight of human epinephrine (adrenaline)?

Ans. 183.207 g/mol

Q.69. What are the other names of adrenaline?

Ans. i) Emergency hormone, and
ii) Flight hormone

Q.70 How many molecules of glucose are released from one molecule of epinephrine?

Ans. About 30,000.

Q.71 From which amino acid epinephrine is synthesized?

Ans. Tyrosine.

Q.72. Which vitamin is required for the synthesis of epinephrine?

Ans. Vitamin 'C'

Q.73 Name the hormone which is responsible for 'fight or flight' response.

Ans. Epinephrine (adrenaline).

Q.74. What is the weight of thyroid gland in a normal adult?

Ans. 20 -25 grams

Q.75. Name some antithyroid compounds.

Ans. Thiourea, thiouracil, PABA, sulfonamides, tolbutamide, sulfadiazine, etc.

Q.76. Name the rate limiting enzyme of catecholamine synthesis.

Ans. Tyrosine hydroxylase.

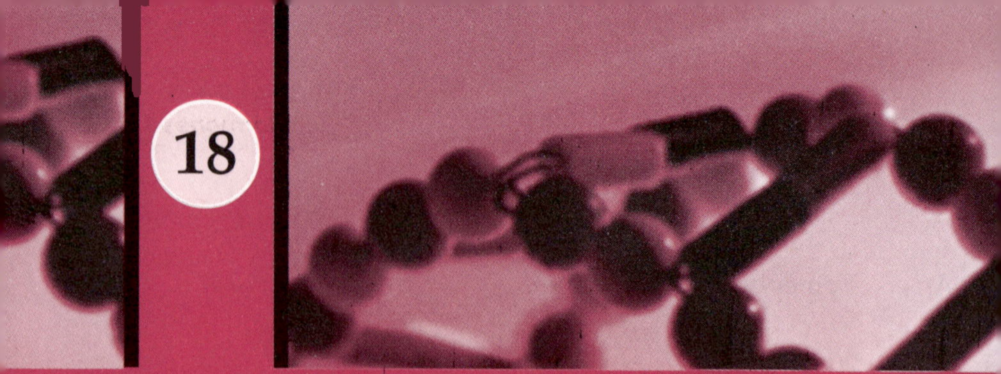

18

URINE/FAECES CHEMISTRY

Q.1. What is the volume of urine excreted per day?

Ans. 1-2 litres

Q.2. What is the principal i.e., main pigment of urine?

Ans. Urochrome

Q.3. What is the normal specific gravity of urine?

Ans. 1.015-1.025

Q.4. Name the preservating agents of urine.

Ans. (i) Toluene,
(ii) Formaldehyde,
(iii) Camphor and
(iv) Thymol

Q.5. What are the normal constituents of urine?

Ans. (i) Water
(ii) Urea
(iii) Uric acid
(iv) Creatinine
(v) Calcium
(vi) Sodium
(vii) Potassium
(viii) Magnesium
(ix) Sulphur (inorganic sulphates, neutral sulphur, conjugated sulphates)

(x) Phosphate
(xi) Ammonia
(xii) Chloride
(xiii) Hippuric acid
(xiv) Oxalic acid, etc.
(xv) Indican
(xvi) Allantoin
(xvii) Purine bases
(xviii) Phenols, etc.

Q.6. Name the organic and inorganic constituents of urine.

Ans.

Organic	Inorganic
1. Urea	1. Chloride as NaCl
2. Uric acid	2. Sodium
3. Creatinine	3. Potassium
4. Hippuric acid	4. Calcium
5. Amino acid nitrogen	5. Magnesium
	6. Phosphorus as phosphates
	7. Sulphur as sulphates

Q.7. What does the specific gravity of urine indicate?

Ans. (i) State of hydration of body
(ii) Concentrating power of kidneys
(iii) Presence of solutes in the urine
(iv) Effect of ADH

Q.8. What is the pH of normal urine?

Ans. 4.3 to 8.0

Q.9. Which apparatus is generally used for determining specific gravity of urine?

Ans. Urinometer

Q.10. Why does the pH of urine increase?

Ans. Due to bacterial conversion of urea to ammonia.

Q.11. Name the conditions in which urine volume gets increased.

Ans. **Physiological conditions:**
(i) Excessive intake of water,
(ii) Excitement,

(iii) Cold climate and
(iv) High protein diet

Pathological conditions :

(i) Diabetes mellitus,
(ii) Diabetes insipidus and
(iii) In certain types of kidney diseases

Q.12. Name the conditions in which urinary volume gets decreased.

Ans. **Physiological conditions:**

(i) In summer or hot weather due to increased loss of water by perspiration.

Pathological conditions :

(i) Fever
(ii) Acute nephritis
(iii) Diseases of the heart and lung
(iv) Diarrhoea and vomiting

Q.13. What are the abnormal constituents of urine?

Ans. (i) Reducing sugars,
(ii) Proteins (mainly albumin),
(iii) Ketone bodies,
(iv) Blood,
(v) Bile pigments (mainly bilirubin) and
(vi) Bile salts

Q.14. Name the conditions in which following abnormal constituents appear in the urine.

Ans.

(i) Glucose	Diabetes mellitus and different types of glucosurias
(ii) Protein	Nephrotic syndrome
(iii) Ketone bodies	Starvation and severe diabetes mellitus
(iv) Blood	Hematuria
(v) Bilirubin	Obstructive jaundice
(vi) Urobilinogen	Hemolytic jaundice

Q.15. What do you understand by the terms 'polyuria' and 'oliguria'?

Ans. If the output of urine excreted is in higher amount than the normal limits, the condition is termed as **'polyuria'** while the decrease in urine output is termed as **'oliguria'.**

Q.16. In which diseases 'polyuria' occurs?

Ans. (i) Diabetes mellitus
(ii) Diabetes insipidus
(iii) Certain diseases of the nervous system
(iv) Contracted kidney
(v) Amyloid degeneration of the kidney and other disorders

Q.17. In which diseases 'oliguria' occurs?

Ans. (i) Acute nephritis
(ii) Diseases of the heart and lungs
(iii) Fever
(iv) Diarrhoea
(v) Vomiting

Q.18. Name the hormone which regulates chloride excretion.

Ans. Aldosterone

Q.19. What is Addison's disease?

Ans. Chronic disease of the adrenal cortex gives rise to Addison's disease.

Q.20. Which hormone remains associated with Addison's disease?

Ans. Aldosterone

Q.21. Why it is called aldosterone?

Ans. Because it contains an aldehyde group at position C_{18}.

Q.22. What is the normal urinary excretion of chloride?

Ans. 10-15 gms of chloride as NaCl

Q.23. In which conditions urinary excretion of chloride gets increased?

Ans. (i) High intake of chloride
(ii) Addison's disease

Q.24. Name the conditions in which urinary excretion of chloride gets decreased.

Ans. (i) Low salt intake
(ii) Diabetes insipidus
(iii) Chronic nephritis
(iv) Diarrhoea
(v) Vomiting
(vi) Cushing's syndrome

Q.25. What is the colour of urine containing bile pigments?
Ans. Yellowish green to brown.

Q.26. By which tests bile pigments in urine may be detected?
Ans. (i) Fouchet's test
(ii) Gmelin's nitric acid test.

Q.27. In which pathological conditions porphyrins are found in the urine?
Ans. Porphyria, which may be either drug induced or due to an inborn error or acquired error of metabolism.

Q.28. What causes benign proteinuria?
Ans. (i) Severe exercise
(ii) Cold bath.

Q.29. What's orthostatic albuminuria /proteinuria?
Ans. It's due to posture, generally upright position i.e. military position.

Q.30. How will you detect protein in urine?
Ans. (i) Heat coagulation test
(ii) Heller's nitric acid ring test
(iii) Sulphosalicylic acid test.

Q.31. How urine is formed?
Ans. It's formed by the following four processes:
(i) Filtration of blood plasma by the glomeruli
(ii) Selective reabsorption of important substances by the renal tubules
(iii) Secretion of certain substances by the tubules
(iv) Exchange of H^+ ions and production of ammonia.

Q.32. Name the hormones involved in the formation of urine.
Ans. (i) Aldosterone
(ii) ADH (antidiuretic hormone).

Q.33. What is the end product of protein metabolism?

Ans. Urea

Q.34. Where does the synthesis of urea occur in the body?

Ans. Liver.

Q.35. What is the daily excretion of urea?

Ans. 20-30 gms.

Q.36. What is the normal level of urea in the blood?

Ans. 14-43 mg%.

Q.37. Which enzyme is responsible to decompose urea to form ammonia?

Ans. Urease.

Q.38. What are the sources of enzyme urease?

Ans. Seeds of:

(i) Watermelon
(ii) Jack beans
(iii) Soyabeans
(iv) Red gram (Arhar dal).

Q.39. What is the normal level of creatinine in blood?

Ans. 0.1-1.2 mg/dl.

Q.40. What is the method by which creatinine is estimated in urine and blood?

Ans. Jaffe's method (Jaffe's reaction).

Q.41. What is creatinine coefficient?

Ans. The number of mg of creatinine excreted daily per kg of body weight is known as the creatinine coefficient.

Q.42. What are the sources of creatine?

Ans. (i) Muscles
(ii) Brain
(iii) Blood etc.

Q.43. In which forms creatine remains present?

Ans. In free or phosphorylated form.

Q.44. What are the precursors of creatine?

Ans. (i) Glycine
(ii) Arginine
(iii) Methionine.

Q.45. What is the normal excretion of creatinine daily?

Ans. 1.0-2.0 g.

Q.46. Name the conditions in which urinary excretion of creatinine is increased.

Ans. (i) Early stages of muscular dystrophy when muscle destruction occurs rapidly.

(ii) In any wasting disease involving increased tissue catabolism

(iii) Hyperthyroidism.

Q.47. Name the renal (kidney) function tests.

Ans. (i) Urea clearance test

(ii) Inulin clearance test

(iii) Creatinine clearance test.

Q.48. Name the actual renal function tests which are in practice these days.

Ans. (i) Estimation of 'urea' level in blood.

(ii) Estimation of 'creatinine' level in serum.

Q.49. What is urea clearance?

Ans. $$\text{Urea clearance} = \frac{\text{mg of urea excreted per minute}}{\text{mg urea per ml of plasma}}$$

Q.50. How will you detect the presence of blood in urine?

Ans. (i) By Benzidine test and

(ii) Orthotolidine test.

Q.51. What do you understand by the words 'Hematuria' and 'Hemoglobinuria'?

Ans. In hematuria one finds the presence of hemoglobin and unruptured RBCs in the urine. It happens when there is some lesion in the kidney or urinary tract.

In hemoglobinuria one finds the presence of hemoglobin only in the urine. It occurs from hemolysis i.e. by the rupturing of the stroma of the RBCs as in the diseases like malaria, typhoid fever, yellow fever, hemolytic jaundice or as a result of the transfusion with incompatible blood.

Q.52. What is the diagnostic importance of Bence-Jones protein found in the urine?

Ans. In cases of:
(i) Multiple myeloma, and
(ii) Myelogenic osteosarcoma.

Q.53. What is "Triple Phosphate"?

Ans. It is Ammonium Magnesium Phosphate.

Q.54. In which disease excretion of calcium in urine is increased?

Ans. Osteomalacia.

Q.55. In which disease excretion of calcium in urine gets decreased?

Ans. Rickets

Q.56. By which test calcium in urine is detected?

Ans. Sulkowitch test

Q.57. In which disease you find increased amount of phenylpyruvic acid in urine?

Ans. In the inherited condition known as "phenylketonuria". In this disorder, phenylalanine is not oxidized to tyrosine due to the absence of an enzyme phenylalanine hydroxylase.

Q.58. Which vegetables contain high amount of oxalic acid/ oxalates or its precursors?

Ans. (i) Asparagus
(ii) Cabbage
(iii) Rhubarb
(iv) Spinach
(v) Tomatoes.

Q.59. Which fruits are rich in oxalic acid/oxalates or its precursors?

Ans (i) Apples
(ii) Grapes
(iii) Lettuce (Chukandar).

Q.60. What is the percentage of glucose in the urine of patients suffering from diabetes mellitus?

Ans. 3 to 5% but may reach upto 10% or even more depending upon the severity.

Q.61. Does the specific gravity of urine decreases or increases in diabetes mellitus?

Ans. Increases.

Q.62. Name the most satisfactory test for the detection of sugar in urine.

Ans. Benedict's test.

Q.63. Name the ketone bodies found in urine.

Ans. (i) Acetone

(ii) Acetoacetic acid

(iii) β-hydroxy butyric acid.

Q.64. By which test ketone bodies are detected in urine?

Ans. Rothera's test.

Q.65. What is Chyluria?

Ans. Chyluria is an abnormality in which the patient excretes milky urine because of the presence of abnormal connection between the urinary tract and the lymphatic drainage system of the intestine, and so-called **Chylous Fistula.**

Q.66. What is the treatment of Chyluria?

Ans. Feeding triacylglycerols in which the fatty acids are of medium chain length (< 12 carbon) in place of dietary fat results in the disappearance of chyluria.

Q.67. Why the urine of those persons is generally reddish-pink who eat beetroot in bulk?

Ans. It is due to the presence of pigments known as **anthocyanins** which remain present in abundance in beetroot. Besides, these pigments are also found in other fruits and vegetables. These pigments are responsible for coloured urines. Such urines superficially resemble that of haemoglobinuria.

Q.68. Name the other vegetables and fruits which are rich in anthocyanins and the individuals eating them pass coloured urines.

Ans. Rhubarb, black berries and binberries.

Q.69. What is the colour of urine in lysol and phenol poisoning?

Ans. It is brownish or black, though it may also sometimes have a greenish tinge in phenol poisoning.

Q.70 What is the colour of the stool in cases of obstructive jaundice?

Ans. Clay-coloured.

Q.71 In which type of disease, faeces in generally, whitish or cream-coloured?

Ans. Pancreatic disease.

Q.72 What is the colour of faeces of those who are on milk-diet?

Ans. Pale yellow or orange.

Q.73 Name the important faecal pigment which generally remains present in it.

Ans. Urobilin (stercobilin).

Q.74. What is the colour of faeces, in whom who eat spinach, and due to which pigment?

Ans. Green, due to the pigment chlorophyll.

Q.75. What do you know about alkaptonuria? What is its formula?

Ans. It this condition, urine darkens upon standing which is due to the conversion of homogentisic acid, the formula of which is as shown below, into substances of unknown composition which are coloured brown or black. This colour also appears in the surface layer. It develops much more quickly in alkaline than in acid urine and comes up within a few seconds when the urine is made alkaline with sodium or potassium hydroxide or with ammonia. This is a difference from melanogen in urine, on which

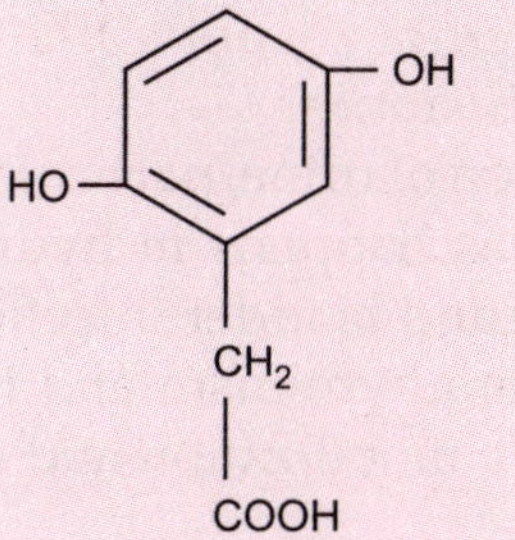

Homogentisic acid

the addition of alkali does not speed-up the oxidation. With melanogen in urine, it is an acid medium which favours the development of the colour.

Metabolism of tyrosine and phenylalanine is defective in this condition so that instead of these substances being completely metabolized, homogentisic acid is formed and excreted in the urine. The condition may be first noticed in early infancy when the napkins are seen to be stained. In later life, cartilages become blackened and may give a bluish tinge to the hollows of the ears and brown colouration of the conjunctiva.

Q.76 Name the other urinary pigments besides urochrome.

Ans. Uroerythrin, uroporphyrin, coproporphyrin, urobilinogen, urorosein, etc.

Q.77. Name the abnormal pigments found in urine.

Ans. Melanin, bilirubin, oxyhaemoglobin, methemoglobin, porphyrins, homogentisic acid, etc.

Q.78 In which disease/disorder melanin is found in urine?

Ans. This type of pigment, never found in urine occurs in patients with melanotic tumours usually when there are secondaries in the liver.

Q.79 Of which substances urinary calculi are formed of?

Ans. Uric acid, urates, calcium oxalate, alkaline earth phosphates (calcium and magnesium), triple phosphate (Magnesium ammonium phosphate), calcium carbonate, cystine and xanthine, Stones of cholesterol, indigo, fibrin and urostealith are very rarely found.

Q.80. Name the factors responsible for the causation of urinary calculi/stones.

Ans.
(i) Stagnation of urine, particularly if there is infection present as happens in hydronephrosis, enlarged prostate and bladder infections.
(ii) Hyperparathyroidism and hypervitaminosis-D
(iii) Excessive mobilization and deposition of calcium.

19

Digestion, Absorption and the Alimentary Tract

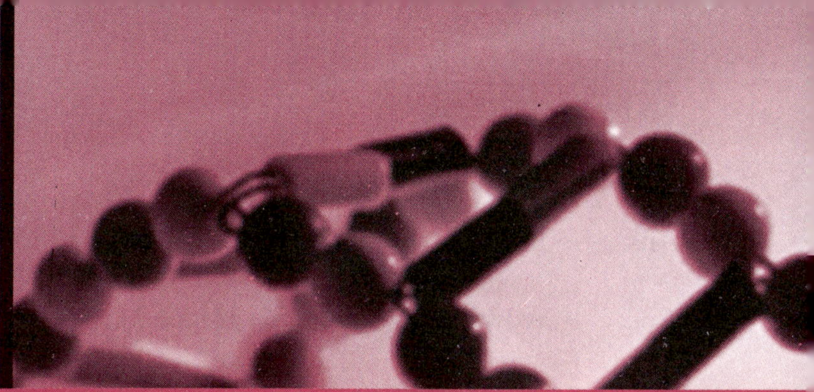

Q.1. What's the action of enzyme ptyalin (salivary amylase)?

Ans. It hydrolyzes starch to maltose.

Q.2. At what pH ptyalin acts?

Ans. 6.8-7.0

Q.3. What's the action of enzyme pepsin?

Ans. (i) It hydrolyzes proteins to proteoses and peptones.
(ii) It also hydrolyzes nucleoproteins to peptones and nucleic acids.

Q.4. At what pH pepsin acts?

Ans. 1-4

Q.5. In which secretion pepsin is found?

Ans. Gastric juice.

Q.6. What is the action of enzyme rennin?

Ans. It hydrolyzes casein to calcium paracaseinate.

Q.7. At what pH rennin acts?

Ans. 1-4

Q.8. What is the function of bile?

Ans. It emulsifies fats, no enzymatic activity.

Q.9. At what pH bile acts?

Ans. 8 -10

Q.10. Where is bile found?
Ans. In liver.

Q.11. What is the action of enzyme trypsin?
Ans. It hydrolyzes peptones to polypeptides.

Q.12. At what pH trypsin acts?
Ans. 8-10.

Q.13. Where trypsin is found?
Ans. It's found in pancreatic juice.

Q.14. What is the action of enzyme pancreatic amylase?
Ans. It hydrolyzes starch and glycogen to maltose.

Q.15. At what pH does pancreatic amylase act?
Ans. 8-10.

Q.16. What is the action of enzyme pancreatic lipase?
Ans. It hydrolyzes fats to fatty acids and glycerol.

Q.17. At what pH pancreatic lipase acts?
Ans. 8-10.

Q.18. What is the action of enzyme enterokinase?
Ans. It hydrolyzes polypeptides to amino acids.

Q.19. At what pH does enterokinase act?
Ans. 8-10.

Q.20. Where is enterokinase found?
Ans. It's found in small intestine **(crypts of Lieberkuhn).**

Q.21. What is the action of enzyme sucrase?
Ans. It hydrolyzes sucrose to glucose and fructose.

Q.22. At what pH does sucrase act?
Ans. 8-10.

Q.23. What is the action of maltase?
Ans. It hydrolyzes maltose to glucose.

Q.24. At what pH does maltase act?
Ans. 8-10.

Q.25. What is the action of enzyme lactase?
Ans. It hydrolyzes lactose to glucose and galactose.

Q.26. What is the action of enzyme lipase?
Ans. It hydrolyzes fats to fatty acids and glycerol.

Q.27. What is the action of enzyme nuclease?

Ans. It hydrolyzes nucleic acids to nucleotides.

Q.28. At what pH enzyme lipase and nuclease act?

Ans. Both between 8-10.

Q.29. Which enzymes are found in intestinal juice?

Ans. Enterokinase, sucrase, maltase, lactase, lipase and nuclease.

Q.30. Which enzymes are found in pancreatic juice?

Ans. Trypsin, pancreatic amylase and pancreatic lipase.

Q.31. What is formed when HCl combines with pepsinogen?

Ans. Pepsin

Q.32. What is the action of rennin?

Ans. Rennin coagulates milk, producing a white mass called curd and a fluid material called whey. The action of rennin is to convert milk proteins, into a form suitable for digestion.

Q.33. By the metabolism of which compound, bile salts are derived?

Ans. Haemoglobin.

Q.34. What is the colour of bile?

Ans. The colour of bile depends upon the type and concentration of pigment that it contains. If the pigment is bilirubin, the bile is yellow, if the pigment is biliverdin, the colour varies from green to black.

Q.35. What are the aftereffects of the removal of gall bladder?

Ans. Removal of the gall bladder diminishes markedly the quantity of bile that will enter the duodenum; therefore, a low fat or non-fat diet is indicated to prevent digestive discomfort.

Q.36. What are the major functions of bile salts?

Ans. (i) Digestion of fats, and

(ii) Absorption of fats

Bile salts act to emulsify the fats into minute fat particles, thus providing a larger surface area for the action of pancreatic lipase.

Q.37. What is pancreatitis?

Ans. It's inflammation of the pancreas which basically involves a lack of coordination between the secretion of pancreatic juice and its ability to flow through the pancreatic duct into the duodenum.

Q.38. What are the plus points of caecum and appendix?

Ans. They serve as store houses for microorganisms which help in digestion. Man cannot digest the complex cellulose found in plant cells without assistance; the stored microbes digest this cellulose for him.

Q.39. What is the length of large intestine?

Ans. 5-6 feet.

Q.40. What is the major function of large intestine?

Ans. (i) Its major function is the reabsorption of water into the body. If all the water in which enzymes are secreted into the digestive tract were lost in the waste material (faeces), man would have a severe problem of dehydration.

(ii) Second function of it is the removal of waste products of digestion (defecation).

Q.41. What is jaundice?

Ans. It is yellowness of the skin and eyes and indicates the presence of bile pigments in the body tissues and a high concentration of bilirubin in the blood.

Q.42. Name the two very important hormones that control the secretory action of the pancreas.

Ans. (i) Secretin, and

(ii) Pancreozymin

Both hormones stimulate the pancreas to secrete its digestive enzymes and alkaline salts.

Q.43. What is metastasis?

Ans. It's spread of cells to other organs.

Q.44. Name the largest glandular organ of the body.

Ans. Liver.

Q.45. What is hepatitis?

Ans. Inflammation of the liver.

Q.46. What is cirrhosis of the liver?

Ans. It is a chronic disease in which the active Kupffer cells are destroyed and replaced by scar tissue. Cirrhosis is commonly associated with repeated episodes of toxic injury or with continuous injury (as in alcoholism) to hepatic cells. Either may lead to progressive fibrous replacement of the damaged cells.

Q.47. What is the main oxidative agent that regulates metabolic rate?

Ans. Thyroxine.

Q.48. What are the main functions of liver?

Ans. Major functions include.

1. **The Production of :**
   (a) Blood/plasma proteins
   (b) Antibodies to fight diseases
   (c) Heparin, a substance that prevents blood clotting, &
   (d) Bile pigments from RBCs in the form of bilirubin and biliverdin.
2. **The storage of :**
   (a) Vitamins and minerals, and
   (b) Glucose in the form of glycogen
3. **The conversion and utilization of :**
   (a) Fats (desaturation), and
   (b) Carbohydrates (glycogenesis)
   (c) Proteins (deamination)
4. **The removal of :**
   (a) Old blood cells and toxins by phagocytosis (Kupffer cells), and
   (b) Waste products (urea and ammonia) from amino acids.

Q.49. What happens when food is oxidized in human body?

Ans. When food is burnt (oxidized) in the system by the cells; sugar, for example, undergoes an oxidation by the cells to produce carbon dioxide, water and energy :

$$C_6H_{12}O_6 + 6O_2 \longrightarrow 6H_2O + 6CO_2 + \text{energy}$$

Q.50. What is the fate of amino acids absorbed in the intestinal tract?

Ans. They are used by the metabolic mill for the :

(i) Synthesis of proteins,

(ii) Are converted to fatty acids, and

(iii) Are converted to glycogen.

OR

(iv) Are oxidized as an energy source.

Q.51. What is the most important role played by amino acids?

Ans. Important role played by amino acids is the donation of their amine group (NH_2), a process called deamination, and transfer of this group to other substances, a process called as transamination.

Deamination and transamination are important in that they are the first step in the metabolic breakdown of these compounds and in the synthesis of amino acids from other compounds.

Q.52. How does cooking influence digestion?

Ans. Cooking significantly improves the digestibility of foodstuffs by the enzymes.

Q.53. What is flatulence?

Ans. It is characterized by increased intestinal motility, cramps and irritation. This occurs due to the indigestion of certain carbohydrates (mostly non-digestible oligosaccharides such as raffinose and leguminous seeds). The di- and oligosaccharides can be metabolized by the intestinal bacteria releasing gases such as hydrogen, methane and carbondioxide, which cause flatulence.

Q.54. What is Hartnup's disease?

Ans. Hartnup is the name of the family in whom the disease was discovered for the first time. It is characterized by the inability of intestinal and renal epithelial cells to absorb neutral amino acids. In this disease, absorption of tryptophan gets most severely affected resulting into symptoms that resemble the patients of pellagra. This is related to the impairment in the conversion of tryptophan to NAD^+ and $NADP^+$, the coenzymes of niacin.

Q.55. What is emulsification and how is it brought about?

Ans It is a process of dispersion of lipids into smaller droplets due to reduction in the surface tension. It is essential for the effective digestion of lipids. Emulsification is brought about by the following mechanisms.

(i) Detergent action of bile salts (glycocholic acid and taurocholic acid).
(ii) Surfactant action of degraded lipids
(iii) Mechanical mixing due to peristalsis

Q.56. How are nucleic acids digested?

Ans. The digestion of nucleic acids takes place in the small intestine. The pancreatic enzymes i.e., ribonucleases and deoxyribonucleases hydrolyze RNA and DNA to oligonucleotides respectively. The latter are degraded by phosphodiesterases to form mononucleotides.
Then, nucleotidases act on nucleotides to liberate phosphate and nucleosides.

Q.57. Name the major disorders of digestion and absorption.

Ans. (i) Peptic ulcers
(ii) Hartnup's disease
(iii) Pancreatitis
(iv) Steatorrhoea
(v) Lactose intolerance

Q.58. What is the length of small intestine in man?

Ans. Nearly 27 feet

Q.59. What are the primary sites of absorption of different things in man?

Ans. Villi

Q.60. How many villi are found in man?

Ans. Nearly five millions

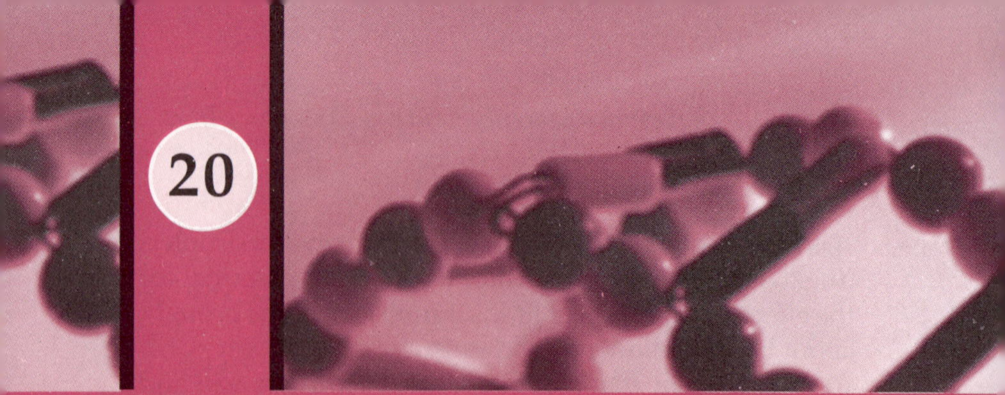

20

Molecular Biology and Genetic Engineering

Q.1. Name the scientist who for the first time synthesized the first artificial DNA gene of yeast.

Ans. Dr. Har Gobind Khorana

Q.2. How many pairs of nucleotides did gene contain which was artificially synthesized by Dr. Har Gobind Khorana?

Ans. 77 (mini gene). The gene synthesized was yeast DNA transcribing transfer RNA alanine.

Q.3. In which year Dr. Har Gobind Khorana was awarded Nobel Prize in Physiology or Medicine and what was his contribution in medical field?

Ans. In the year **1968** along with **Nirenberg** & **Holley**. He interpreted the genetic code and its function in **protein synthesis**.

Q.4. What do you understand by 'Southern Blot'?

Ans. It is a technique for 'Blot Transfer'; since this technique was designed and developed by the scientist **Southern**, hence the name to this technique is given '**Southern Blot**'. In this technique, the cut-bits of DNA (item 1) are separated by agarose or polyacrylamide gel disc electrophoresis, denatured and transferred to nitrocellulose paper. Then, the paper is exposed to c-

DNA (complementary DNA) probe which hybridizes with complementary fragments in the filter. With the exposure to X-ray, the DNA fragments that recognized and hybridised with the c-DNA probe are identified.

Q.5. What do you understand by 'Northern Blot' technique?

Ans. In this case, the RNA is subjected to electrophoresis followed by blot transfer. The identification of a specific RNA molecule is achieved by the use of labelled complementary DNA (c-DNA) probe.

The hybrids formed between RNA and c-DNA can be identified by radioautography.

Q.6. What is restriction fragment length polymorphisms (RFLPs)?

Ans. The human genome is heterogenous, containing slight variations in base sequences (usually once in every hundred base pairs) that differ from individual-to-individual, but may not generally affect the structure and function. **These differences in the DNA structure are referred to as restriction** fragment polymorphisms (RFLPs) that can be examined by cleaving DNA into fragments by restriction endonucleases.

Q.7. What are the uses of RFLPs?

Ans. RFLPs are useful for the diagnosis of molecular diseases for e.g. sickle cell anaemia. In forensic medicine, **RFLPs serve as DNA finger-prints for the identification of criminals or in setting the dispute of parenthood. This is done by using 'Southern Blot Technique'.**

Q.8. What is Western Blot Technique?

Ans. This is a technique for the identification of a specific protein. The mixture of proteins is subjected to electrophoresis, transferred to nitrocellulose and then probed by using a labelled antibody probe.

Q.9. What do you understand by the term 'blotting techniques'?

Ans. The analytical techniques used for the identification of specific DNA, a RNA or a protein from thousands of each are collectively referred to as blotting techniques.

These are :

(i) **Southern Blot** (for DNA)

(ii) **Northern Blot** (for RNA), and

(iii) **Western Blot** (for protein)

Southern blot technique is named after the name of the scientist who identified it while the other two names are laboratory jargons (unfamiliar words) which are now accepted.

Q.10. Name the scientist responsible for inventing PCR technique and in which year.

Ans. This method for the first time was invented in **1984** by the scientist **Dr. Kary Mullis** which permits the synthesis of millions of copies of specific DNA sequence in a few hours. The source of target DNA may be from animal, plant, bacterium or virus.

Q.11. Was Dr. Kary Mullis awarded Nobel Prize, if yes, in which year?

Ans Yes, in the year **1993**

Q.12. What are the applications of PCR?

Ans. Due to the speed and specificity in the amplification of target DNA molecules, PCR has distinct advantages over the other traditional methods of recombinant DNA technique. PCR is highly sensitive, it can detect even the presence of a single molecule of DNA. PCR has several applications as in the :

(i) Rapid diagnosis of infectious diseases like AIDS, tuberculosis, Hepatitis B, C, etc.

(ii) Prenatal diagnosis of genetic diseases

(iii) Detection of criminals in forensic medicine, and

(iv) Study of evolution from DNA of archaeological samples.

Q.13. What is polymerase chain reaction (PCR)?

Ans. It is a novel test tube technique of DNA amplification which is capable of producing millions of copies in hours with ease, accuracy, specificity and sensitivity.

Q.14. What is the usage of PCR?

Ans. It has revolutionized genetic engineering for making human life more comfortable as regards diseases and in agricultural sciences also for hybrid variety etc.

Q.15. What is recombinant DNA technology?

Ans. The genetic manipulations in the laboratory involving the isolation and cloning (making identical copies) of a specific DNA are collectively referred to **as recombinant DNA technology or more commonly genetic engineering.**

Q.16. Name the scientists who developed recombinant DNA technology for the first time.

Ans. It was first developed by **Paul Berg, Herbert Boyer and Stanley Cohey in 1973.**

Q.17. Which stages are broadly involved in recombinant DNA technology?

Ans. Following stages are broadly involved :
(i) Isolation of a specific DNA
(ii) Selection of vectors
(iii) Preparation of chimeric DNA and
(iv) Cloning of the chimeric DNA

Q.18. How many restriction enzymes have been isolated so far from different organisms?

Ans. **About 400**

Q.19. What is a vector?

Ans. A vector is a carrier of DNA molecule to which the fragment of interest (say a human gene) is attached for cloning. The essential preparation of a vector includes its ability for autonomous replication, the presence of a specific nucleotide sequence recognized by a restriction endonuclease and a gene for identification.

Q.20. Name the types of vectors which are commonly used in recombinant DNA technology.

Ans. Three types namely :
(i) Plasmids
(ii) Bacterophages, and
(iii) Cosmids

Q.21. What are plasmids?

Ans. Some of the bacteria contain small, independent circular double stranded DNA molecules known as plasmids. They provide resistance to the bacteria against antibiotics. Plasmid DNAs replicate independently and they can be easily separated from the host bacteria. The DNA sequences and restriction maps (characteristic of endonuclease action) of many plasmids are known. This is useful for the incorporation of foreign target DNA into the vector. Plasmids, the most commonly used vectors can accept DNA fragments of 6-10 kilobase (kb) length.

Q.22. What are bacteriophages?

Ans. These are linear DNA molecules, containing several restriction enzyme sites. They can accept foreign DNA fragments of 10-20 kb length (kilo base - a unit designating the length of a nucleic acid sequence, e.g., 1 kb = 1,000 nucleotide long base sequence).

Q.23. What are cosmids?

Ans. These are specialized plasmids containing DNA sequence namely Co-sites. Cosmids have got the capability to accept much longer DNA fragments (20-50 kb).

Q.24. What are DNA probes?

Ans. DNA libraries contain thousands or sometimes millions of DNA fragments, therefore, it is extremely difficult to choose a DNA sequence of interest from among these. A group of molecules, namely DNA probes are used to search the libraries for specific genes or c-DNAs. The probes are usually single stranded pieces of DNAs (sometimes RNAs), labelled with the radioisotopes such as ^{32}P. The probes containing complementary base sequence are used to identify specific DNA fragments of DNA libraries. The Southern and Northern blot techniques respectively identify DNA and RNA by use of probes.

Q.25. What is a genomic library?

Ans. A genomic library is prepared from the partial digestion of total DNA of a genome by the use of restriction endonucleases. These DNA fragments may be ligated to a vector to produce recombinant DNA molecules that can replicate in the host bacteria. The amplified DNA fragments representing the genome of a particular species constitute a genomic library.

Q.26. What is a complementary DNA library?

Ans. c-DNA library contains only copies of DNA sequences that are present in the mRNA molecules. These are prepared from the mRNA which serves as a template to prepare a complementary double stranded DNA (c-DNA) using the enzyme reverse transcriptase. c-DNA libraries contain relatively smaller DNA fragments compared to genomic libraries.

It is estimated that the genomic library of E.coli has about 30,000 DNA fragments while that of man has about one million DNA fragments.

Q.27. What do you understand by DNA libraries and what are their types?

Ans. The collection of genetic fragments constitutes DNA libraries which are mainly of two types, namely; (i) genomic library, and (ii) cDNA library.

Q.28. How is recombinant DNA or chimeric DNA prepared?

Ans. The main purpose of genetic engineering is to insert a DNA of interest into a vector DNA so that the DNA fragment replicates along with the vector. The hybrid combination of two fragments of DNA is referred to **as recombinant DNA or chimeric DNA** (chimera is a monster in Greek mythology that has a lion's head, a goat's body and a serpent's tail. This may be compared to Narasimha in Indian mythology).

A fragment of target DNA (from human) and the vector DNA (from plasmid) produced by a specific restriction endonuclease, possessing sticky ends, can be conveniently used for the preparation of recombinant DNA. The human DNA and vector DNA with complimentary sequences are annealed. The enzyme, namely DNA ligase ligates (seals) the DNA fragments to finally produce recombinant DNA as shown below (Fig 1).

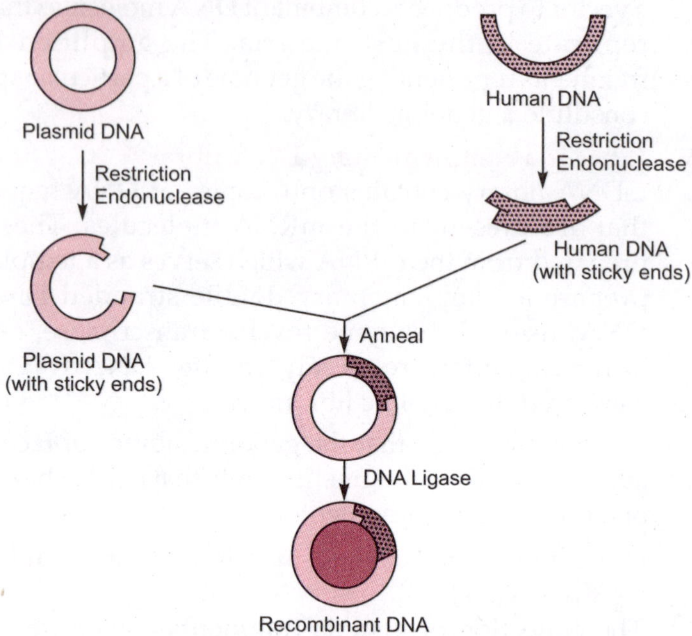

Fig. 1: To show diagrammatic representation of the production of a recombinant DNA molecule.

For the ligation of two DNA fragments, sometimes a synthetic DNA called a linker is used. The linker helps for the recognition of human DNA and vector DNA (particularly with blunt ends).

Q.29. Name some genetic disorders for which DNA probes are now available.

Ans. (i) Cystic fibrosis
(ii) Tay-Sachs disease, and
(iii) Duchenne's muscular dystrophy, etc.

Q.30. What do you understand by the cloning of the recombinant DNA?

Ans. A clone means a large population of identical copies. These may be molecules, cells or bacteria that are derived from a common ancestor. The recombinant DNA contained in a plasmid (vector) can be easily introduced into bacterial cells by a process called transformation. The replicating bacterial cell permits the amplification of the recombinant DNA of the vector. In this way, cloning results in the production of large number of identical target DNA molecules (Fig 2). The cloned target DNA is then released from its vector by cleavage (using appropriate restriction endonucleases), isolated, characterized and used for various purposes.

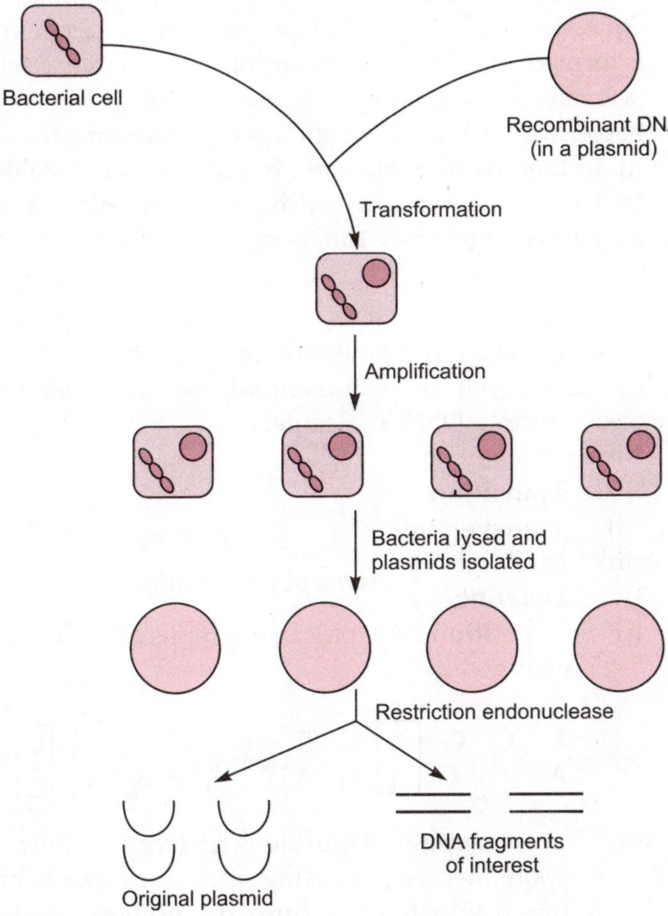

Fig. 2: To show cloning of a recombinant DNA

Q.31. What is a gene?

Ans. It's the biological unit of heredity. It is the sequence of a DNA molecule specifying one complete polypeptide chain. Biochemically, it is called a cistron. Gene in prokaryotes may be a continuous unique sequence of nucleotides and the DNA may be polycistronic i.e., transcribes more than one mRNA producing different proteins/enzymes but the eukaryote cistron (gene) may be discontinuous in the DNA molecule as exons are separated by introns. After transcription the introns-transcripts are excised out and the exons-transcripts spliced to give the mRNA proper. Only a single mRNA is formed and hence the eukaryote DNA is monocistronic. A virus may contain only a dozen genes while a bacterium several thousands genes. **Human genome has up to 1.5 million gene pairs but only about 1,00000 (one lakh) are involved in coding for proteins.** The others may have regulatory functions.

Q.32. What is mutation in a DNA molecule (genes)? Explain with suitable examples.

Ans. Mutation is a replacement of nitrogen base with another in one or both the strands or addition or a deletion of a base pair in a DNA molecule.

Mutation may be:

(i) **Transition**
(ii) **Transversion**
(iii) **Insertion** } **Frame shift mutation**
(iv) **Deletion** }

(i) **Transition :** AT pair being replaced by GC pair changed to

T C G [A] C T   T C G [G] C T
A G C [T] G A changed to A G C [C] G A

(ii) **Transversion:** A purine is replaced by pyrimidine spontaneously or using analogues like 5–bromo-uracil which substitutes thymine or cytosine in course of replication of DNA.

e.g. Adenine being replaced by thymine

T C G [A] C T   T C G [T] C T
A G C [T] G A changed to A G C [A] G A

Transversion may be :

(a) **Non-detectable:**
For e.g., Hb A with alanine at B67 in place of valine. No change in the function if alanine replaces valine, e.g., (Hb Sydney).

(b) **Missense effect :** (i) Acceptable, Hb A lysine B 61 and Hb Hikari B 61 asparagine (ii) partially acceptable, Hb A (B 6 glutamate) and Hb S (B 6 valine), (iii) Unacceptable Hb A (58 hist), Hb M (58 tyrosine).

(c) **Non-sense effect:** Premature termination of protein synthesis; amino acid sequence is garbled (dressed) for e.g. Hemoglobinopathies.

(iii) **Insertion** (frame shift mutation): A new pair is introduced. Chemicals like acridine can be introduced non-covalently.

(iv) **Deletion** (frame shift mutation): A pair can be deleted by loss of purines on hydrolysis, alkylation, deamination, etc. U.V., gamma rays and X-rays can also cause deletion. Proflavin effects cross-linking and deletion.

Q.33. What is Pol III* star (Pol III*)?

Ans. **Arthur Kornberg (father)** claimed that his DNA polymerase was the enzyme required for the synthesis of DNA but **later on, his son, T. Kornberg corrected his father's statement** by publishing that it is the DNA polymerase III enzyme which is involved in the synthesis of DNA and what his father had, was different, i.e. it was DNA polymerase I which can only do the repair of defective DNA but is unable to synthesize it. Obviously, father got disturbed over his son's contradiction and found that DNA polymerase III of his son was also not the enzyme involved in the synthesis. He found that biologically active form is a dimer of Pol III which he (A. Kornberg) called Pol III* star. He also showed that Pol III* should have a cofactor of Co Pol III* and it is the complex of Pol III* and Co Pol III* that initiates and does the synthesis of DNA.

Q.34. What do you understand by recombinant DNA, natural DNA and artificial DNA?

Ans. **Recombinant DNA:**

Combinations of portions of DNA from one molecule to another in the same cell or cell of one species to another yield recombinant DNA. Such combinations may be : (i) natural and (ii) technological. If it is technological and deliberately produced, it becomes recombinant DNA technology (genetic engineering).

Natural DNA:

Natural recombination of DNA could be between (a) molecules of DNA: (b) homologous chromosomes.

DNA combinations can occur between:

(i) Virus and virus
(ii) Virus and bacteria
(iii) Bacterium and bacterium, and
(iv) Bacterium and eukaryotes.

Artificial DNA (Recombinant DNA)

In the experimental procedure, the primer DNA is purified and mixed with digested plasmid DNA both of which having been treated with restriction enzymes and incubated at low temperature of 10-15, so that, the complementary strands are joined together by H–bonds. The gaps are sealed by DNA ligase. The plasmid with recombinant DNA is introduced into a calcium shocked bacterium and amplified. In this way artificial recombinant DNA is produced.

Q.35. Who produced synthetic DNA for the first time and by which means?

Ans. **For the first time, synthetic DNA was produced by the scientist Dr. Har Gobind Khorana by chemical means.** Short segments (10-15 nucleotides) with sticky ends were synthesized chemically. With T_4 ligases, these were connected to give synthetic DNA with sticky ends.

Q.36. What is the approximate DNA content of cells and viruses of different species?

Ans. The DNA content of cells of different species is as mentioned below:

Species	DNA (μg per cell as virion). values are for eukaryotes for somatic (diploid cells).	Number of nucleotide pairs in millions (x 10^6)
Amphibian	7	6500
Mammals	6	5500
Higher plants	2.5	2300
Fishes	2	2000
Birds	2	2000
Fungi	0.02-0.17	20
Bacteria	0.002-0.6	2
Bacteriophage (T_4)	0.00024	0.17
Bacteriophage lambda	0.00008	0.05

Q.37. What is recombinant DNA technology and genetic engineering?

Ans. Recombinant DNA technology and genetic engineering means **"gene synthesis and transferring"** which confer upon us :

(i) Some pains,
(ii) Some tears,
(iii) Some cheers, and
(iv) Some gains.

It takes one thorn out of chest of man and shapes another thorn to take the test of man. Therefore, guidelines had to be issued to genetic engineers not to engineer recombinants which increase fears. Recombinant DNA technology in genetic engineering which effects artificial modifications of the genetic constitution of a living cell by introducing a foreign DNA through experimental techniques. DNA fragments of different origins are joined with the help of enzymes chiefly restriction endonucleases and DNA ligases and such recombinant DNA of host parasite DNA an amalgamation is introduced into appropriate hosts say E. coli which is cloned. The recombinant DNA having the desired gene replicates, transcribes and translates. A gene of choice can be combined to give a desired precious biochemical like growth hormone or insulation.

Various biological tools of recombinant technology are :

(i) The enzymes,
(ii) Passenger DNA, and
(iii) Vehicle DNA

It is the bacteria which have given the wonderful enzymes, the restriction endonucleases for selective scission of DNA molecules for tailoring, the exonucleases, reverse transcriptase, DNA polymerase, DNA ligase etc.

It is again the bacteria which have donated plasmids for functioning as vehicles (bacteriophages, e.g., bacteriophage lambda are also used as vehicle).

It is again bacteria which are impregnated with the recombinant DNA to be delivered as a full-grown metamorphosed baby-DNA of choice. Passenger DNAs include (a) complementary DNA (cDNA), (b) synthetic DNA, and (c) random DNA.

Q.38. What are the plus and negative points (repercussions) of recombinant DNA technology and its future?

Ans. **Following are the important plus points:**

1. Because of the development of Recombinant DNA Technology, there would be better understanding of the living systems and the life.
2. **Production of Enzymes :** Genes could be used for bulk production of enzymes for use in laboratory and industry.
3. **Production of Insulin :** As one knows, the disease **Diabetes Mellitus** is on increase **World over,** therefore, there is greater and greater demand for insulin for its treatment. By this technique, insulin is produced these days commercially on large scale.
4. There could be better understanding of gene expression for e.g. in arresting the growth of cancer by regulating gene expression.

5. **Production of Interferons :** Recombinant DNA technology would go a long way in the production of adequate amount of interferons for therapeutic purposes.
6. **New antibiotics :** New antibiotics or improved ones from the existing antibiotics can be prepared.
7. **Growth hormone :** If growth hormone somatotrophin and its release inhibiting factor somatostatin are to be prepared from life sources only, then half a million sheep brain are to be used to get just a few milligrams. Genetic engineering litres of bacterial culture without sacrificing the animals.
8. **Production of Ethylene glycol :** It is in great demand for industry. Preparation of the same from ethylene is made possible by this technology.
9. **Production of Energy :** Many of the fuels are hydrocarbons. Microorganisms can be produced by this technique to convert desert plants into hydrocarbon-producing ones for catering to the energy needs.
10. **Mosquito, fly and bug menace :** Special strains of microbes which could totally destroy mosquitoes, flies and bugs can be thought of to **make earth the heaven for the humans and the cattles.**
11. **Curing of Inborn-Errors :** By the development of this kind of technology, there is great hope that the inborn errors of metabolism could be cured by introducing the required gene(s) through viruses like polyoma, SV-40 in replacement of defective genes **by gene replacement therapy.**
12. **Solution to pollution problems :** New strains of microbes **capable of eating away oil wastes,** harmful natural gases and industrial spits could be created.
13. **Good and improved food :** Good quality food and increased yield of crops is now possible by applying this technology and revolution in this

field is coming slowly by which no one on earth is expected to remain hungry. Incorporation of **'nif genes'** to cereals has given much higher yield of the crops.

14. **Sequence analysis of DNA :** Cloning for sequence analysis is helpful in unravelling the molecular mysteries and to think of having only good genes in a person by tailoring.
15. **Gene Banks, etc. :** Gene banks and libraries for research in molecular biology and biotechnology (in case of humans/animals and plant kingdom), getting for e.g. superman and everything super whether in case of animal kingdom or plant kingdom are the upcoming benefits of recombinant DNA technology.

Recombinant DNA technology is not a bed of Roses alone but a bed of thorns as well which may produce unending hazards etc. for the 'creation'.

Negative points are:

(A) If, by any chance, in the course of cloning using bacterial vectors some drug resistant and at the same time harmful bacteria are let loose into the world, these new creations may cause incurable diseases to the humanity and the live stock. An unanticipated epidemics could be spread-out to utmost danger. It is suggested that (i) the plasmids should be of non-transmissible type and should not have genes coding for drug resistance and (ii) only certain plasmids should be used and the release of organisms with recombinant DNA to the environment should be strictly forbidden.

(B) In case pathogens having cancer - causing gene say a polyoma virus or those which could cause typhoid or diarrhoea are let loose, genetic engineers would be doing a disservice to humanity perhaps to a great measure and on experimental explosions.

(C) By creating genes of choice, the healthy division of living systems as prokaryotes and eukaryotes may be lost ushering in a catastrophic ecological imbalance.

(D) There is a craze among the scientists to work only in the **field of recombinant DNA technology as it is a fertile field for harvesting Nobel Prizes** but it is suggested that **Nobel Prize** should not be given to the contributors in the field of genetic engineering. **The extremists like George Wald of Harward, Nobel Laureate and others** have observed that "the recombinant DNA technology" confronts our society with problems unprecedented not only in the history of science but also of the life on earth. But there are two sides of the coin as in the case of a razor blade, fire, electricity or atomic power. **Man should use this technology only to make heaven but not hell.**

Q.39. How is human insulin produced commercially these days by recombinant DNA technology?

Ans. **Scientist Robert Crea** and his group at California have succeeded in synthesizing human insulin who adopted the method of Khorana and Itakura. Applying Khorana's method, DNA with the sequence known for A and B was synthesized and inserted separately into two RBR 322 plasmids by the side of β–galactosidase gene, the recombinant plasmids were separately incorporated into E.coli cells. The bacteria secreted fused β–galactosidase A and B chains. They were separated by HPLC. By Crea's phosphtriester synthetic technology and purification by HPLC, insulin is prepared these days commercially on large scale.

Q.40. What are unwindase and rewindase in DNA transcription?

Ans. Separate enzymes to unwind DNA remain present for replication of DNA for the formation of RNA from DNA template **(transcription),** the enzyme DNA directed unwinds and rewinds the DNA and is said to have **unwindase and rewindase activity.**

Q.41. What will happen if a severe diabetic takes insulin by mouth instead of injection?

Ans. Insulin being a protein will be digested **by proteinases, peptidases,** etc. to amino acids, if taken by mouth. **Net result is nil.**

Q.42. What is NUDIKI?

Ans. It is an enzyme called as Nucleoside Diphosphokinase catalyzing the interconversion of ATP, GTP, CTP and TTP.

$$\text{GTP + ADP} \xrightarrow{\text{NUDIKI}} \text{GDP + ATP}$$

Q.43. Name the enzymes that can relax or insert supercoils.

Ans. (i) Topoisomerases
(ii) Gyrases

Supercoiling is seen in most naturally occurring DNA molecules.

Q.44. How many nucleotide base pairs are found in human diploid genome?

Ans. About 7×10^9 nucleotide base pairs.

Q.45. What would be the length of human diploid genome if its nucleotide base pairs are placed end-to-end?

Ans. About three meters long.

Q.46. What are proto oncogenes?

Ans. They are normal genes, but when activated become active oncogenes.

Q.47. What are pseudogenes?

Ans. These are inactive genes but have DNA sequences resembling normal genes.

Q.48. What is the full form of DNAP?

Ans. DNA polymerase.

Q.49. How many types of polymerases are found in bacteria?

Ans. Three, i.e.:
(i) DNAP I (ii) DNAP II and
(iii) DNAP III

Q.50. How many types of DNA polymerases are known in eukaryotes?

Ans. Five types i.e.:

(i) DNAP alpha

(ii) DNAP beta

(iii) DNAP gamma

(iv) DNAP delta and

(v) DNAP epsilon

Q.51. What is Kornberg's enzyme? Who discovered it? Was he awarded Nobel Prize?

Ans. Kornberg's enzyme is DNA polymerase I. Arthur Kornberg discovered it by isolating it from Escherichia coli in 1956 for which he was awarded **Nobel Prize in 1959.**

Q.52. What do you know about DNAP I?

Ans. It is a single polypeptide (103 KD), which is mainly a repair enzyme. It has both $3' \rightarrow 5'$ and $5' \rightarrow 3'$ exonuclease activities. When $5' \rightarrow 3'$ exonuclease domain is removed, the remaining fragment (68 KD) retains the polymerization and proof reading activities; it is then known as **Klenow fragment**. This enzyme is widely used in recombinant DNA technology.

Q.53. What is the main function of DNAP III?

Ans. It is the main replication enzyme in bacteria. It has a molecular weight of 900 KD and has a proof reading ability.

Q.54. What is the function of bacterial DNAP II?

Ans. Bacterial DNA polymerase II (88 KD) has 4 subunits and is used for:

(i) DNA repair and

(ii) Proof reading

Q.55. What is the main function of eukaryotic (mammalian) DNAP alpha?

Ans. This enzyme is mainly responsible for chromosome replication. This enzyme has got the capability to polymerize about 100 nucleotides per second. Contrarily, bacterial enzymes polymerize about 1000 nucleotides per second.

Q.56. What is primosome?

Ans. The regulatory apparatus for lagging strand synthesis is called **primosome which consists of 7 different proteins, including helicase, protein C and primase.** The primosome moves along the lagging strand in 5' → 3' direction.

Q.57. What is the effect of Etoposide in mammalian topoisomerases?

Ans. Mammalian topoisomerases are inhibited by etoposide, and therefore, it is commonly **used as an anticancer drug.**

Q.58. What are the main characteristics of mammalian DNA polymerase?

Ans. These are as mentioned below :

DNAP	Alpha	Beta	Gamma	Delta	Epsilon
Location	Nucleus	Nucleus	Mitochondria	Nucleus	Nucleus
Function	Lagging strand synthesis	Repair of leading strand	Replication	Leading strand synthesis	Repair of lagging strand
Primase Activity	Yes	No	Yes	No	No
3'→5' exonuclease	No	No	Yes	Yes	Yes
Proof Reading Activity		Main enzyme	15%	15%	

Q.59. How many enzymes and proteins do participate in DNA replication?

Ans. More than 20 enzymes and proteins do participate which are collectively called as DNA replicate system or replisomes.

Q.60. Does the DNA synthesis require RNA primer?

Ans. Yes, the initiation of DNA synthesis requires RNA primer, about 10-200 nucleotide long. This RNA is synthesized by a RNA primase (molecular weight 60 KD).

Q.61. What are Okazaki fragments?

Ans. The small DNA molecules attached to its own primer RNA are called Okazaki fragments.

Q.62. What is Xeroderma pigmentation (XP)?

Ans. It was originally described by **Moritz Kaposi in 1882**, is a rare autosomal recessive condition in which DNA repair mechanisms are defective. DNA damage produced by UV irradiation, especially thymine dimers, cannot be excised in this condition. Main clinical symptom is the sensitivity to UV rays; with sunlight causing blisters in the skin which leads to hyperpigmentation and atrophy of skin. Death usually occurs in the second decade of life due to squamous cell **carcinoma of skin.**

Q.63. What is Ataxia-telangiectasia?

Ans. It is an autosomal recessive disease. In this disease, increased sensitivity to UV and X-ray is observed. Cerebellar ataxia and lymphoreticular neoplasms are common in this condition. Ataxia-telangiectasia mutated (ATM) gene has been isolated. It has been found to remain present in 1% of total population and has been found **in the ratio of 1:40,000 persons** who inherit 2 copies of the ATM alleles.

Q.64. Name the other diseases of genetic defects in DNA repair.

Ans. These are :

(i) Bloom's syndrome,

(ii) Progeria,

(iii) Fanconi's anemia,

(iv) Cockayne's syndrome, and

(v) Hereditary polyposis colorectal cancer **(HPCC or Lynch syndrome).**

In Bloom's syndrome, chromosomal breaks and rearrangements are noticed and DNA ligase-I is found to be defective. The condition is manifested by facial erythema, photosensitivity and telangiectasia.

Progeria, though rare is also believed to be due to defective DNA repair in which ageing process is so **rapid**

that a 6 year old child looks to be 60 years old and dies at a young age.

Q.65. What do you understand by telomere?

Ans. The replication always takes place from 5' → 3' direction. In the lagging strand, the replication process is by formation of small pieces (Okazaki pieces). Therefore, a small portion (about 300 nucleotides) in the 3' end of the parent strands can not be replicated. This end piece of the chromosome is called **telomere.**

Q.66. What is telomerase?

Ans. The continuous shortening of telomere end is prevented by an enzyme called as **telomere terminal transferase or telomerase**. This enzyme synthesizes (TTAGG) in repeats on to the telomere sequence. To this extended region in the lagging strand, DNA primase and DNA polymerase act to produce an okazaki piece and thus shortening of chromosome is prevented. Tremendous work has been done on telomerase **by Shipper in 1990.**

Q.67. How many do mammalian cells contain DNA dependent RNA polymerases (RNAP) and what are their functions?

Ans. Mammalian cells do contain 3 different DNA dependent RNA polymerases. Their molecular weight ranges from 500,000 to 600,000.

RNAP type I or A is responsible for the synthesis of rRNA. RNAP type II or B is responsible for the synthesis of almost all mRNAS. It is inhibited by **alpha amanitin** (a toxin found in the mushroom **Amanita phalloides).** RNAP type III or C is responsible for the production of t—RNA.

Q.68. What are ribozymes?

Ans. Enzymes made-up of RNA are called ribozymes. **This recent finding has changed the general concept that all enzymes are made-up of proteins.**

Q.69. Who discovered Ribozymes?

Ans. **Thomas Cech and Sidney Altman** discovered the ribozymes for which they were **awarded Nobel Prize in the year 1989.**

Q.70. How many transcription initiation sites are generally present in the entire DNA of human beings?

Ans. About 1,00000.

Q.71. What is the action of antibiotic Actinomycin D obtained from streptomyces upon the synthesis of RNA?

Ans. It inhibits the synthesis of RNA by inserting phenoxazone ring between two G-C bp of DNA template.

Q.72. What is the action of antitubercular/antileprotic drug upon the synthesis of RNA?

Ans. It inhibits the synthesis of RNA by binding rifampicin to beta subunit of RNA polymerase which gets inactivated.

Q.73. What is the action of alpha amanitin (α-toxin) obtained from mushroom upon the synthesis of RNA?

Ans. It inhibits the synthesis of RNA by inactivating RNA polymerase II.

Q.74. What is the half life of mammalian m-RNA?

Ans. Few hours, but some have only few minutes.

Q.75. What is the effect of estradiol upon the half-life of m-RNA?

Ans. It prolongs it from few hours to about 200 hours.

Q.76. What about the m-RNA synthesis in mature RBCs?

Ans. Since, in the mature RBCs, the nucleus is deleted, therefore, there is no new m-RNA synthesis.

Q.77. What about the protein synthesis in mature RBCs?

Ans. Since the metabolism of mature RBCs is also minimal, therefore, protein synthesis is also less.

Q.78. What type of virus is human immunodeficiency virus causing AIDS?

Ans. Retrovirus in which a single stranded DNA is produced by the enzyme, RNA dependent DNA polymerase or reverse transcriptase.

Q.79. Who isolated for the first time reverse transcriptase enzyme?

Ans. **Temin and Baltimore** for which they were awarded **Nobel Prize in 1975.**

Q.80. What do you understand by transfer RNAs?

Ans. They are RNA molecules present in the cytoplasm. Each molecule is only 73-93 nucleotides in length, much shorter than the m-RNA molecules. Since they are easily soluble, they are also referred to as soluble RNA or s-RNA. The transfer RNA reveals extensive internal base pairing and acquires a clover leaf like structure.

Q.81. What are the structural features of t-RNA molecule?

Ans. A unique feature of t- RNA when compared to other RNA molecules is that they contain a significant proportion of unusual bases, for instance:

(a) Dihydrouracil,
(b) Pseudouridine,
(c) Ribothymidine, and
(d) Inosine, as well as methylated bases.

Besides, the 5' end often has a phosphorylated guanosine.

Q.82. What is ribosomal RNA (r-RNA)?

Ans. Ribosomal assembly is the protein synthesizing machinery.

Q.83. What are small nuclear RNAs (sn-RNAs)?

Ans. Their size ranges, from 90 to 300 nucleotides and may present about one million copies per cell. Some of them like U_1, U_2 and U_5 are involved in spliceosomes for intron removal. U_4 is used for poly-A processing.

Q.84. Who deciphered (interpreted hidden writings) the genetic code for the first time? What do you know about genetic code?

Ans. **Nirenberg** was awarded **Nobel Prize in 1968 for deciphering genetic code.** By trial and error it was first established that the codon for each amino acid was a triplet sequence of nucleotides on the m-RNA. Since there are 4 different bases, they can generate 64 (4^3) different codons or code words by permutation (variation in the order of things) and combinations. **Matthaei and Nirenberg** after establishing the existence of the triplet codon, tried to decipher the codon for each amino acid.

Q.85. What are punctuator codons or terminator codons (Non-sense codons)?

Ans. There are the following three punctuator codons or terminator codons, namely:

(i) UAA,
(ii) UAG, and
(iii) UGA

These do not code for any particular amino acid and were first known as "nonsense codons" **but are now more correctly termed as punctuator codons or terminator codons.**

Q.86. What is the chain initiator codon for almost majority of polypeptide chains?

Ans. **AUG** acts as the initiator codon for most of the polypeptide chains synthesized but for a few cases, **GUG** may also act as the initiating codons.

Q.87. How many t-RNAs are found in mitochondria?

Ans. Approximately 22

Q.88. How many peptide bonds are synthesized per minute by one ribosome?

Ans. Approximately 100

Q.89. What is the difference between polyribosomes and polysomes?

Ans. No difference.

Q.90. What is the literal meaning of chaperone?

Ans. Chaperone literally means elderly lady-in-charge of unmarried girls on social occasions.

Q.91. What are the examples of chaperones?

Ans. Examples of chaperones are a large family of proteins called **heat shock proteins (HSPs)** which were for the first time identified in response to heat shock.

Any stress to the cell including toxins, heavy metals, bacteria, radiation, free radicals, etc. will cause increased production of HSPs, and hence they are more correctly termed as **stress proteins.** They are highly conserved throughout evolution. They also facilitate the correct fate of the proteins, such as their assembly, or controlled switching between active or inactive conformations. The concentration of **HSP** is increased when protein synthesis gets increased as in cell division or recovery from toxicity or during malignant transformation.

Q.92. What is the classification of chaperones?

Ans. They are classified into 4 major families such as:
(i) HSP - 10
(ii) HSP - 60
(iii) HSP - 70
(iv) HSP - 90
The numbers representing the molecular weight in KD.

Q.93. Where does remain locate the gene for HSP-70 and on which chromosome?

Ans. The gene for HSP-70 remains located within the major histocompatibility complex on the short arm of chromosome number 6.

Q.94. What is the main function of HSP-60 (Chaperonin) and HSP-70 classes?

Ans. The main functions of them is to stabilize unfolded or partially folded polypeptides and to facilitate the correct fate of the proteins. Be it known that proteins have to perform a variety of very important functions in human body.

Q.95. Does abnormal folding of proteins unassisted by chaperones lead to any disease?

Ans. It leads to :
(i) Alzheimer's disease, and
(ii) Prion disease

Q.96. How many nucleotides are expected to be found in mitochondrial DNA?

Ans. About 16,500.

Q.97. For the synthesis of how many ribosomal RNAs, t-RNAs and proteins does DNA contain information within it?

Ans. (i) 2 ribosomal RNAs,
(ii) 22 t-RNAs, and
(iii) 13 proteins
All the above are components of ETC (electron transport chain).

Q.98. How do antibiotics tetracyclins, streptomycin, erythromycin, etc. inhibit the protein synthesis? How does diphtheria toxin act?

Ans. It's as follows :

Name of the antibiotic	Action
1. **Tetracyclins**	Inhibit t-RNA binding to ribosomes.
2. **Streptomycin** (was isolated by **Selman Waksman in 1940,** who got **Nobel Prize in 1952)**	Causes misreading of codons, hence nonfunctional proteins are synthesized.
3. **Erythromycin**	Translocation is inhibited.
4. **Mitomycin** (used as anticancer drug)	It intercalates with DNA strands, thus blocking transcription and translation as well as replication.
5. **Actinomycin** (used as anticancer drug)	It inhibits m-RNA synthesis.
Name of the toxin	**Action**
1. **Diphtheria toxin,** an exotoxin liberated by the bacteria coryneba - cterium diphtheria.	It causes inactivation of EF-2 by covalent attachment of ADP to EF-2 and inhibits protein biosynthesis in mammalian systems (Eukaryotes)

Q.99. Give one example of the diseases of mitochondrial myopathies.

Ans. Leber's hereditary optic myopathy.

Q.100. What are the characteristics of Leber's hereditary optic myopathy?

Ans. It's characterized by blindness in young males more often than in females. The disease is transmitted maternally. It is caused by a single base mutation which alters an arginine codon to histidine codon in NADH coenzyme Q reductase.

Q.101. Who is said to be 'Father' of heredity?

Ans. **Gregor Johann Mendel** (1822-84).

Q.102. In which year Gregor Johann Mendel described the principles of heredity?

Ans. 1865.

Q.103. Give some examples of the diseases of autosomal dominant inheritance.

Ans. They are:

(i) Chondrodystrophy (a type of dwarfism)
(ii) Aniridia (absence of iris)
(iii) Neurofibromatosis,
(iv) Epiloia (skin rash + epilepsy) and
(v) Some types of porphyrias, etc.

Q.104. Give some examples of sex-linked recessive inheritance.

Ans. (i) Hemophilia
(ii) Glucose-6-phosphate dehydrogenase deficiency,
(iii) Pseudohypertrophic muscular dystrophy (Duchenne type), and
(iv) Red-green colour blindness, etc.

Q.105. How abnormal genes can be identified?

Ans. These can be identified by the advanced techniques of DNA hybridization with gene probes. Diagnosis may also be done in utero by taking cells by amniocentesis, and probing with such genes.

Q.106. How the treatment of genetic disorders is possible?

Ans. This may be done at different levels, for e.g.:

(i) Replace the end product of the missing enzyme, e.g. administer thyroxine in familial goiter.
(ii) Limit the substrate of the missing enzyme. In phenylketonuria, reduce phenylalanine in the diet. In galactosaemia, remove lactose from the diet.
(iii) Replace missing protein, administer AHG in haemophilia.
(iv) Increase the activity of abnormal enzyme, e.g. large quantities of vitamin B_{12} is useful in methylmalonic aciduria.

(v) Induce the enzyme; in **Crigler Najjar Syndrome**, the activity of enzyme **glucuronyl trasferase** can be induced by the drug phenobarbitone.

(vi) Gene therapy is still in experimental stage but may become common in the next generation.

Q.107. Who is the Director of Human Genome Project?

Ans. At present **Francis Collins** who is also director of the National Institute of Health (NIH) in Bethesda, U.S.A. **He is known for his notable discoveries of disease genes.**

Q.108. How many genes are found in human beings?

Ans. **About 20,000-25,000** (as per the latest discovery of Human Genome Project)

Q.109. How many base pairs are found in total DNA of a human?

Ans. **About 3 billion base pairs** which reside in the 23 pairs of chromosomes within the nucleus of all our cells.

Q.110. What is the location of genes in human chromosomes?

Ans. A small list is as mentioned below:

Location		:	Gene
Chromosome	1	:	Alkaline phosphatase (liver, bone, kidney)
	1	:	Salivary amylase
	1	:	Apolipoprotein A-II
Chromosome	2	:	Alkaline phosphatase (placental)
	2	:	Apolipoprotein - B
	2	:	Immunoglobulin, Kappa chain
	2	:	Pro-opiomelanocortin
Chromosome	3	:	Transferrin
Chromosome	4	:	Alcohol dehydrogenase
	4	:	Alpha fetoprotein
	4	:	Fibrinogen
	4	:	Interleukin-2
	4	:	Huntington's chorea (disease)

Chromosome	5	:	HMG CoA reductase
Chromosome	6	:	Steroid-21, hydroxylase
	6	:	MHC (Major histocompatibility) locus
Chromosome	7	:	Urea cycle enzymes
	7	:	Cystic fibrosis (disease)
Chromosome	8	:	Carbonic anhydrase
	8	:	Thyroglobulin
Chromosome	9	:	Interferon
Chromosome	11	:	Haemoglobin β, γ and δ chains
	11	:	Proinsulin
	11	:	Pepsinogen
	11	:	Parathyroid hormone
Chromosome	12	:	α-2 - macroglobulin
	12	:	Glyceraldehyde-3-P-dehydrogenase
Chromosome	13	:	Adenosine deaminase
Chromosome	14	:	Immunoglobulin heavy chains
	14	:	α_1 - antitrypsin
Chromosome	15	:	Cytochrome P-450
Chromosome	16	:	Haemoglobin α-chain
	16	:	Adult polycystic kidney disease
Chromosome	17	:	Growth hormone
	17	:	RNA polymerase II
Chromosome	18	:	Prealbumin
Chromosome	19	:	Carcinoembryonic antigen
	19	:	β-chain of HCG
	19	:	Creatine phosphokinase, M-chain
	19	:	LDL receptor
Chromosome	20	:	Adenosine deaminase
Chromosome	21	:	Superoxide dismutase

Chromosome	22	:	Immunoglobulin, lambda chain
Chromosome	X	:	Glucose-6-P-dehydrogenase
	X	:	Antihemophilic globulin
	X	:	HGPRTase
	X	:	Duchenne type muscular dystrophy (disease)
	X	:	Ornithine transcarbamoylase
Chromosome	Y	:	Steroid sulfatase

Q.111. What is point mutation?

Ans. Mutations occur when changes take place in the nucleotide sequences of DNA molecule. Single base changes are called **point mutations.**

Q.112. What is transition?

Ans. Transition is where a pyrimidine base is changed to another pyrimidine (e.g. T to C) or a purine is changed to another purine (e.g. A to G).

Q.113. What is transversion?

Ans. If a purine is changed to a pyrimidine (e.g. A to C) or a pyrimidine to a purine (e.g. T to G), it is called a transversion.

Q.114. What is p^{53}? What do you know about it?

Ans. It is an oncosuppressor protein which is referred to as the **"molecule of 1993"** because a large number of papers were published on p^{53} in a single year. It has a molecular weight of 53 KD and has 393 amino acids. Its half-life is only 5-10 minutes. It inhibits cell division, allowing them to repair, or leading to **PROGRAMMED CELL DEATH (APOPTOSIS).**

Q.115. Name the scientist who is pioneer in genetic recombination studies.

Ans. Bacterial genetic studies give us much insight into the switching of genes. **Severo Ochoa** is the pioneer in genetic recombination studies who was awarded **Nobel Prize in 1959 for his tremendous fascinating work in recombinant DNA technology which is the need of the day.**

Q.116. What is repression and induction?

Ans. The synthesis of functional proteins such as enzymes is generally controlled by the process of **repression and induction.**

Some genes are expressed constitutively i.e. their product proteins are always seen in appreciable quantity inside the cell. On the other hand, some genes are inducible, which means that they are expressed in response to an inducer.

Q.117. How many diseases have a genetic basis?

Ans. More than 3,000

Q.118. Define cell signalling.

Ans. In multicellular organisms there is a need for the cells to communicate with one another in order to co-ordinate their growth and metabolism. The main way by which cells communicate with each other is by means of extracellular signalling molecules or hormones. These molecules are synthesized and secreted by signalling cells and produce a specific response in target cells that have specific receptors for the signalling molecules. Different cells can respond differently to the same signalling molecule depending upon the type of receptor and the intracellular reactions initiated.

Q.119. What is the classification of cell signalling?

Ans. Cell signalling can be classified into three distinct types based on the distance over which the signalling molecule acts. (a) **in endocrine signalling**, the signalling molecule (e. g. insulin) acts on target cells distant from the site of synthesis in cells of an endocrine organ (e.g. the pancreas). The endocrine cells secrete the signalling molecule into the blood stream which carries it to the target cells elsewhere in the organism. (b) **In paracrine signalling**, the signalling molecule affects only target cells close to cell from which it was secreted. The communication from one nerve cell to another by chemical neurotransmitters is an example of paracrine signalling. (c) **In autocrine signalling,** where a cell responds to a molecule that it has produced itself.

Q.120. What is G-protein?

Ans. G-protein (G for guanyl nucleotide) is a signal–coupling protein. Its main function is in signal transduction; besides it also stimulates the activity of adenyl cyclase, an enzyme that increases the concentration of cAMP (second messenger) by forming it from ATP. Second messenger plays very important role in many ways.

Q.121. What are G-protein linked receptors?

Ans. On binding, its ligand a G-protein ligand receptor activates G proteins [guanyl nucleotide (GTP) binding proteins] which, in turn, activate or inhibit either an enzyme that generates a specific second messenger or an ion channel, causing a change in the membrane potential. Epinephrine and glucagon act through interaction with G-protein linked receptors. The majority of G-protein – linked receptors contain seven transmembrane α – helices. Thus, they have a similar overall shape to that of bacteriorhodopsin (which is not a receptor). G-proteins remain localized in the cytosolic face of the plasma membrane and act as an-off molecular switches. When it has guanosine diphosphate (GDP) bound, the G-proteins in the 'off' state. The activated receptor causes it to release the GDP and exchanges it for GTP, converting it to the 'on' state. The activated G-protein with its bound GTP then dissociates from the receptor and binds to and activates an effector enzyme (e.g. adenylate cyclase) which, in turn, catalyzes the formation of a second messenger (e.g. c-AMP). The G-protein then hydrolyzes the bound GTP, causing it to revert back to the 'off' state. Cholera toxin acts by inhibiting the intrinsic GTP are activity of the G-proteins with the result that once activated to the GTP-bound state the G-protein can not be turned off again.

Q.122. What are second messengers?

Ans. The binding of ligands to many G-protein linked receptors leads to a short-lived increase in the concentration of certain intracellular signalling molecules called second messengers. (the hormone/ligand can be considered as the first messenger). **The major second messengers include:**

(a) 3′, 5′ - cyclic AMP (**c-AMP**),
(b) 3′, 5′ - cyclic GMP (**c-GMP**),
(c) Inositol 1, 4, 5 – triphosphate (**IP_3**),
(d) 1, 2 – diacylglycerol **(DAG)**, and
(e) **Ca^{2+}**

The elevation in the level of one or the other of these second messengers then leads to a rapid alteration in cellular function. c-AMP and c-GMP are derived from ATP and GTP by the actions of adenylate cyclase and guanylate cyclase, respectively. For example, the action of glucagon on glycogen metabolism is mediated through the second messenger c-AMP. IP_3 and DAG are derived from the membrane lipid phosphatidylinositol 4,5,-biphosphate (which is a phosphorylated derivative of phosphatidylinositol) by the action of phospholipase C which is also located in the plasma membrane and like adenylate cyclase, is activated by G-proteins. One of the main actions of the polar IP_3 is to diffuse through the cytosol and interact with Ca^{2+}channels in the membrane of the endoplasmic reticulum, causing the release of stored Ca^{2+} ions which, in turn, mediate various cellular responses. The DAG produced by the hydrolysis of phosphatidylinositol 4, 5-diphosphate, along with Ca^{2+} ions released from the ER (endoplasmic reticulum), activates proteins kinase C, a membrane bound enzyme that phosphorylates various target proteins, again leading to alterations in a variety of cellular processes.

Q.123. Who worked out the three dimensional structure of DNA?

Ans. In 1953, Scientists Watson and Crick worked out the three dimensional structure of DNA, starting from X-ray diffraction photographs taken by other two scientists, namely Franklin and Wilkins.

Q.124. What do you know about Radial loops?

Ans. When chromosomes get depleted of histones, they are seen to have a central fibrous 'protein scaffold' to which the DNA is attached in loops, therefore, *in vivo* it seems likely that the next order of packaging involves the attachment of the 30 nm fibre to multiple locations on the central protein scaffold in a series of radial loops. Little is known as to how this structure is organized.

Q.125. In which infectious diseases, polymerase chain reaction (PCR) based diagnosis is helpful?

Ans. It's helpful in the following infectious diseases; i.e.,

(i) HIV (ii) Tuberculosis

(iii) Hepatitis A, B, C, D and E

Q.126. In which haematological disorders, PCR based diagnosis is helpful?

Ans. It's helpful in the following haematological disorders; i.e.:

(i) Lymphoma

(ii) Haemophilia

(iii) Leukaemia

Q.127. In which genetic disorders, PCR based diagnosis is helpful?

Ans. It's helpful in the following genetic disorders; i.e.:

(i) Fragile X-syndrome

(ii) Muscular dystrophy

Q.128. In which type of cancers, PCR based diagnosis is helpful?

Ans. It's helpful in the following types of cancers; i.e. :

(i) Neuroblastoma

(ii) Sarcoma

(iii) Thyroid carcinoma

Q.129. What is a gene?

Ans It's a biological unit of heredity. It is the segment of a DNA molecule specifying one complete polypeptide chain. Biochemically, it is called a cistron.

Gene in prokaryotes may be a continuous unique sequence of nucleotides and the DNA may be polycistronic, i.e., transcribes more than one in RNA producing different proteins/enzymes. Side-by-side, eukaryotic cistron (gene) may be discontinuous in the DNA molecule as extrons are separated by introns.

Q.130. How many gene pairs are found in human genome and how many of them are involved in coding for protein?

Ans It has up to 1.5 million gene pairs, out of which only about one lakh are involved in coding for proteins, whereas the others may have regulatory functions.

Q.131. Name the various 'biological tools' of recombinant technology.

Ans (1) Enzymes
(2) Passenger DNA, and
(3) Vehicle DNA

Foreign DNA which is passively transferred from one cell to another cell or organ is known as the passenger DNA while the DNA which acts as the carrier as the vehicle DNA.

Q.132. Can Kornberg's enzyme i.e. DNA polymerase repair the damaged DNA?

Ans. No.

Q.133. By which enzyme damaged DNA can be repaired?

Ans. Polynucleotide ligase

Q.134. What is another name of DNA polymerase?

Ans. DNA nucleotidyltransferase.

Q.135. What is the full name of Kornberg?

Ans. Arthur Kornberg

Q.136. In which year Arthur Kornberg discovered the enzyme DNA polymerase?

Ans. 1957

Q.137. What are the main functions of nucleases?

Ans. (i) They are required for the repair of damaged DNA
(ii) They are required for genetic recombination
(iii) They are also probably required for the complex process of DNA replication.

Q.138. What is Central Dogma of Molecular Biology?

Ans. Francis Crick had formulated what came to be known as the Central Dogma of Molecular Biology, namely, that information could flow from DNA to RNA to protein (DNA ⟶ RNA ⟶ protein) but could not flow backward from protein to either RNA or DNA (protein ↛ RNA ↛ DNA). In June, 1970, Baltimore and quite independently, Howard Temin announced the discovery of an enzyme reverse transcriptase or RNA—directed DNA polymerase, which is capable of transcribing RNA into DNA as shown below:

$$\text{RNA} \xrightarrow[\text{transcriptase}]{\text{reverse}} \text{DNA}$$

Apparently certain viruses, like the RNA tumour viruses used by Baltimore, could produce DNA from a RNA template. For this work Baltimore shared Nobel Prize in 1975 along with Temin and Dulbecco.

Q.139. What do you know about the chemistry and role of nitric oxide (NO) in the humans?

Ans. It is another signalling molecule, which neither needs vesicular transport for secretion, nor does it need any receptor at the target cell. It diffuses through plasma membrane and plays a vital role:

(i) In the vasodilation (dilation of blood vessels).
(ii) Its deficiency causes angina.
(iii) It plays vital role in the control of viral/bacterial infection.
(iv) It plays role in the neurotransmission (including penile erection).

The work on the role of NO as a signalling molecule was recognized in 1998 by the award of Nobel Prize for Medicine to the three scientists of U.S.A., namely Robert F. Furchgott, Louis J. Ignarro and Ferid Murad.

Q.140. What are ras Genes?

Ans. The ras genes were first identified as those responsible for the tumorigenic properties of the Harvey (H-ras) and Kirsten (K-ras) sarcoma viruses, which produce tumors in animals and provided the first evidence that cellular counterparts in human cells might be involved in the development of human tumors. The **ras gene** products are proteins located at the inner face of the plasma membrane. They bind to guanine nucleotides and function as molecular switches that regulate mitogenic signals from growth factors to the nucleus via signal transduction pathways.

Q.141. What are c-myc Genes?

Ans. The c-myc gene, located on chromosome 8, is the protooncogene of avian myelocytoma virus. It binds to DNA and is involved in transcription regulation. The gene product, p 62 is located in the nucleus of transformed cells and levels of c-myc correlate with the rate of cell division.

Q.142. How many genetic disorders are known today in humans?

Ans. About 6,000 genetic disorders.

Q.143. Does a normal person contain a mutated gene(s)?

Ans. Each one of us has **5-50** mutated genes that could have serious consequences depending upon the circumstances.

Q.144. What are the plus points of finding diseased-gene(s)?

Ans. Finding of diseased gene(s) enables one to predict those who are at risk even before they develop the illness, or those whose children might be at risk even before the conception.

Q.145. What do you understand from the term monogenic diseases?

Ans. These result from modifications in a single gene occurring in all cells of the body.

Q.146. Name 10 unusual genetic mutations (disorders) in humans which are very rare.

Ans.

Sl. No.	Unusual genetic mutation	Repercussion
1	**Progeria**	Causes accelerated aging. Most children of this disease die of age-related diseases around the age of 13.
2.	**Uner Tan Syndrome**	Sufferers of this disease walk on all fours **(quadru-**

		pedal locomotion) and have a congenital brain impairment. **UTS** is a syndrome that was proposed by the Turkish evolutionary biologist **Üner Tan** after studying 5 members of the Ulas family in rural Turkey
3.	**Hypertrichosis** (Werewolf synd-rome or Ambras Syndrome)	Sufferers have **excessive hair** on the shoulders, face, and ears. Studies have implicated it to a rearrangement of chromosome 8.
4.	**Epidermodysplasia Verruciformis**	Sufferers are prone to widespread human papillomavirus (HPV) infection. This infection causes scaly macules and papules (cutaneous squamous cell carcinomas) to grow on the hands, feet and even face. These skin **'eruptions'** appear as wart-like lesions- & even wood- like and horn-like growths- with reddish - brown pigmented plaques.
5.	**Severe combined Immunodeficiency Disorder (SCID)**	It's a disorder in which individuals are born without any effective immune system.

6.	**Lesch-Nyhan Syndrome**	**LNS** is a genetic disorder that affects one in every 380,000 births, nearly all of them boys. **It results in an overproduction of uric acid.** Such patients release excess uric acid through their blood which builds-up under the skin causing **gouty arthritis.** It can also cause **kidney and bladder stones.** The disease also affects neurological functions and behaviour. Individuals exhibit involuntary body movements, like tensing muscles, jerking movements & self-mutilating behaviours (damage their own organs/parts of the body by biting off the tips of their own fingers or bite their lips).
7.	**Electrodactyly** (formerly known as **"lobster claw hand"**	Such patients suffer from **split-hand/split-foot malformations** which are rare limb deformities which can manifest in any number of ways.
8.	**Proteus syndrome**	It's a condition in which bones, skin and other tissues are overgrown. Individuals typically have organs and tissues that grow out of proportions

		with the rest of their body resulting in strange and inbalanced features.
9.	**Trimethylaminuria (Fish odor syndrome)**	This disorder is very rare and very obvious when someone with **trimethylaminuria** is standing next to you. Individuals with the condition, because they cannot break down the naturally occurring but pungent smelling-trimethylamine, **literally smell like rotting fish, rotting eggs, garbage or urine. Trimethylaminuria** is found in sweat, urine, exhaled breath and other bodily secretions.
10.	**Marfan's syndrome**	It's a disorder of the connective tissues. People with the syndrome tend to have long and thin arms and legs. Syndrome causes bones to overgrow and create loose joints. Overgrown ribs can cause the chest bone to bend inward or push outward. **Spinal curvature** is another problem.

Q.147. Name most common genetic diseases (disorders) of humans.

Ans.

S. No.	Genetic Disease	Cause(s)
1.	**Cystic fibrosis**	One of the most widespread inherited disorders. It results when lack of certain protein is present and the balance of chloride in the body is not restricted. Symptoms include difficulty in breathing, recurrent lung infections, digestive and reproductive issues. It occurs only when both parents are carriers.
2.	**Severe Combined Immunodeficiency Disorder (SCID)**	As its name suggests, this disorder affects functioning of immune system. This disorder is caused by the mutation of more than one gene and renders a person unable to fight off any kind of infection (germs). It's believed to be caused by the absence of, or lack of **Adenosine deaminase (ADA),** as well as notable defects in T and B cell responses.
3.	**Tay-Sachs disease**	**Tay-Sachs** disease causes death at an early age, usually around 5 years,

		because of the absence of enzyme **Hexosaminidase-A**. Progressive destruction of the nervous system & the brain takes place in this disease. There is no treatment, only management of the symptoms.
4.	**Jackson-Weiss Syndrome**	This syndrome is caused by a premature **fusion of the bones of the skull (irregularly shaped skull),** which leads to the deformity of the head and face and also mental retardation and crossed eyes (abnormal placement of the eyes), a bulging forehead and foot abnormalities. Anyone with this disorder usually lives a normal lifespan.
5.	**Fragile-X Syndrome**	Fragile-X, a group of genetic conditions, affects families differently. The syndrome causes inherited mental disabilities. Fragile-X- associated tremor/ataxia syndrome affects those with high testosterone and fragile X-associated primary ovarian insufficiency affects those with ovaries.

6.	**Sickle cell disease (SCD)**	It is an inherited disease where the RBCs, normally shaped like discs, instead form a crescent or sickled shape. This reduces the RBCs ability to carry oxygen to all the tissues of the body-which can result in painful sickle cell crisis & can occur for just a few times in a person's life or many times. Besides pain (abdominal, chest and bones), other symptoms include fatigue, shortness of breath, increased heart rate, delayed growth & puberty. **Treatment :** Stem cell transplant is the only available treatment which is used only in severe SCD, otherwise daily intake of antibiotic along with extra folic acid is recommended. **Blood transfusion is a usuful treatment for some situations.**
7.	**Thalassemias**	The thalassemias (β-thalassemia is the most common, **α-thalassemia is less common**) is a group of inherited blood disorders where, hemoglobin, the oxygen carrying molecule, is not properly synthesized by the red blood cells which

results in an anemia - where the usual symptoms are fatigue, an enlarged spleen, easily broken bones, bone pain and shortness of breath. People with thalassemia may also have poor appetite, darkened urine and jaundice, frequent infections, etc.

Q.148. Give a list of specific genetic disorders.

Ans.
1. Autism
2. Autosomal Dominant Polycystic Kidney disease
3. Breast Cancer
4. Colon Cancer
5. Cystic fibrosis
6. Down syndrome
7. Duchenne Muscular Dystrophy
8. Familial Hypercholesterolemia
9. Fragile X syndrome
10. Gaucher's disease
11. Hemochromatosis
12. Hemophilia
13. Huntington's disease
14. Klinefelter's syndrome
15. Marfan's syndrome
16. Neurofibromatosis
17. Osteogenesis imperfecta
18. Parkinson's disease
19. Phenylketonuria
20. Poland syndrome
21. Porphyria
22. Porgeria
23. Prostate cancer
24. Sickle cell disease
25. Skin cancer
26. Spinal Muscular Atrophy
27. Tay-Sachs disease
28. Thalassemias
29. Trimethylaminuria
30. Turner's syndrome
31. Wilson's disease

21

CANCER BIOCHEMISTRY

Q.1. What is Cancer?

Ans. Cancer is characterized by the following three main properties, viz;

(i) Unrestricted growth

(ii) Invasion on local tissues; and

(iii) Spread or metastasis to other parts of the body

Q.2. Which type of cancer is the largest killer?

Ans. Breast

Q.3. Name some clinically useful tumour markers and their associated cancer(s).

Ans.

	Marker	Associated Cancer
1.	Carcinoembryonic antigen (CEA)	Colon, lung, breast, pancreas
2.	Human chorionic gonadotropin (HCG)	Trophoblast, germ cell
3.	Alpha-fetoprotein (AFP)	Liver, germ cell
4.	Calcitonin (CT)	Thyroid (Medullary carcinoma)
5.	Prostatic acid phosphatase (PAP)	Prostate

Q.4. For which type of cancer, the detection of Bence-Jones protein in urine is meant?

Ans. Multiple myeloma and myelogenic osteosarcoma.

Q.5. What is carcinogenesis?

Ans. The substances/agents causing cancer are known as carcinogens and the phenomenon is known as carcinogenesis. These carcinogens may either be exogenous or endogenous in nature.

Q.6. What are co-carcinogens?

Ans. These are the substances which have got the capability to activate/induce the carcinogens. **Methylcholanthrene** for instance can cause carcinoma of the skin at a very high concentration but if **croton oil** is mixed with it, then it may cause skin cancer at a very low concentration. In this case, croton oil acts as a co-carcinogen, hence termed as a co-carcinogen.

Q.7. What is the classification of carcinogens?

Ans. They have been placed in the following four categories/groups:

(i) Chemical compounds, for e.g., benzidine, 2-naphthylamine, asbestos, nickel compounds, 4-nitrophenyl, cigarette's smoke, chromium compounds, tar, etc.

(ii) Endocrine factors, e.g. estrogens and androgens.

(iii) Oncogenic viruses, e.g., papova group viruses and leukoviruses, and

(iv) Ionizing radiations, e.g., ultraviolet rays.

Q.8. What is metastasis?

Ans. It's the spread of cancer cells from a primary place of origin to other tissues where they grow as secondary tumours, and it's the major problem presented by this disease (cancer).

Q.9. What is the comparison of rate of oxygen consumption of cancerous cells versus normal cells?

Ans. Rate of consumption of oxygen of cancerous cells is somewhat less than the normal cells.

Q.10 What is the comparison of the utilization of glucose of cancerous cells versus normal cells?

Ans. Malignant cells tend to utilize from **5 to 10 times** more glucose than the normal cells and convert most of it to lactic acid.

Q.11. What is the difference in the pH of a cancerous tissue versus normal tissue?

Ans. pH of cancerous tissue is about 7.0 as compared to 7.4 of a normal tissue.

Q.12. What are the salient enzymatic features of cancerous cells?

Ans. Cancerous cells exhibit the following salient features :

1. Low (↓) levels of enzymes, i.e.,
   (a) Cytochrome oxidase,
   (b) Succinic dehydrogenase
   (c) D-amino acid oxidase, etc.
2. Raised (↑) levels of enzymes, i.e.,
   (a) Nucleases,
   (b) Arginase,
   (c) Xanthine oxidase
   (d) β-glucuronidase
   (e) Certain peptidases,
   (f) Glycolytic enzymes, etc.
3. Rate of oxygen consumption of cancerous cells is somewhat less than the normal cells.
4. **Malignant cells utilize 5–10 times more glucose** than the normal cells and convert most of it to lactic acid.
5. Several malignant tumours have been found to have **high levels of glycolytic enzymes** and the necessary cofactors i.e., (phosphate and nicotinamide dinucleotide.
6. Role of aldoreductases in such cells is of considerable importance.

Q.13. What are the various important types of antitumor agents?

Ans. These are as given below:

a) **Alkylating agents,.** for e.g., mephalan, cyclophosphamide, busulfan, etc.
b) **Nucleic acids inhibitors,** for e.g., 6-mercaptopurine, 6-thioguanine, 8-azaguanine, aminopterin, amethopterin, etc.
c) **Plant alkaloids,** for e.g., vincristine, vinblastine, etc.
d) **Antitumor antibiotics,** for e.g., actinomycin-D, mitomycin-C, mithramycin, adriamycin, etc.
e) **Hormonal agents,** for e.g., estrogens, androgens, progestins, thyroxine, etc.
f) **Immunotherapy**: Effective in cutaneous melanoma (cancer of skin)

Q.14. Name the radioactive isotopes which are generally used in the treatment of cancer i.e., in radiation therapy.

Ans. Cobalt–60, Cesium–137, Radium–226 etc.

Q.15. What are the hazards of radiation therapy?

Ans. It is known to be mutagenic, carcinogenic and teratogenic and has been found to be associated with an increased risk of developing both secondary leukaemias and solid tumours.

Q.16. Is there any relation of excess intake of calories versus cancer?

Ans. Excess intake of calories may be correlated to some extent with increased risk of cancer.

Q.17. What is mutation?

Ans. Unusual changes in cell division is known as mutation.

Q.18. What are mutagens?

Ans. Substances which can cause mutation are known as mutagens. Risk of cancer is greater on exposure to these mutagens.

Q.19. Name some mutagens which are generated upon storage of food.

Ans. (i) Malonaldehyde,
(ii) Mycotoxins, and
(iii) Fumigation products, etc.

Q.20 Name some mutagens which are generated during food processing.

Ans. (i) Products of heating

(ii) Smoking, broiling (cooking on coal),
(iii) Irradiation. (iv) Solvent extraction, etc.

Q.21. Name some mutagens which are used as food additives.

Ans. (i) Food colours,
(ii) Food flavours,
(iii) Preservatives,
(iv) Sweetners, and
(v) Antioxidants, etc.

Q.22 Name some natural food constituents which act as mutagens.

Ans. (i) Flavonoids,
(ii) Furans and
(iii) Alkaloids

Q.23. Whether vegetarians or non-vegetarians are prone to cancer?

Ans. Epidemiological studies have shown that vegetarians have lower risk of cancer than the non-vegetarians because of the fact that green coloured raw vegetables possess antimutagens and anticarcinogens in abundance which include methylated flavonoids, aromatic isothiocyanates, coumarins, plant sterols, protease inhibitors, ascorbic acid, tocopherols, retinols, etc.

Q.24. Name the anticancerous agents/phytochemicals present in tomato, papaya, carrot, strawberry and apricot.

ans. (i) Vitamin C, and
(ii) Lycopene

Q.25. Name the anticancerous agents/phytochemical present in chillies.

Ans. Capsenin

Q.26 Name the anticancerous agents/phytochemical present in water melon and citrus fruits respectively.

Ans. Carotenoids (especially cantalop) and limonin respectively.

Q.27. Name the anticancerous agents/phytochemical present in tea leaves and carrots respectively.

Ans. Polyphenols and β-carotene respectively.

Q.28. Name the anticancerous agents/phytochemical present in cauliflower, cabbage, radish and mustard.

Ans. Indole–3–carbinol

Q.29. Name the anticancerous agents/phytochemical present in soyabean, groundnut and germinating alfa–alfa.

Ans. Gentisin

Q.30. Name the anticancerous agents/phytochemical present in garlic and onion.

Ans. Allicin

Q.31. What is DNA chip?

Ans. A thumb–nail sized chip containing an array of upto 30,000 short DNA sequences; used mostly in research to discover new tumour markers.

Q.32. What is cancer staging?

Ans. The process by which cancer is divided into groups of early and late disease; useful for prognosis and helps guide therapy selection.

Q.33. What is prostate–specific antigen (PSA)?

Ans. A kallikrein–like serine proteinase produced by epithelial cells of both benign and malignant prostate tissue.

Q.34. What is a tumour marker?

Ans. A substance found in an increased amount in the blood, other body fluids, or tissues that may suggest the presence of a type of cancer.

Q.35. Which organs/tissues are most vulnerable for cancer?

Ans. It's as mentioned below in decreasing order:

(a) Breast,
(b) Prostate,
(c) Lung,
(d) Colon–rectum, and
(e) Bladder

Q.36. Name the main anticancerous agents/phytochemical present in carrots.

Ans. β-carotene

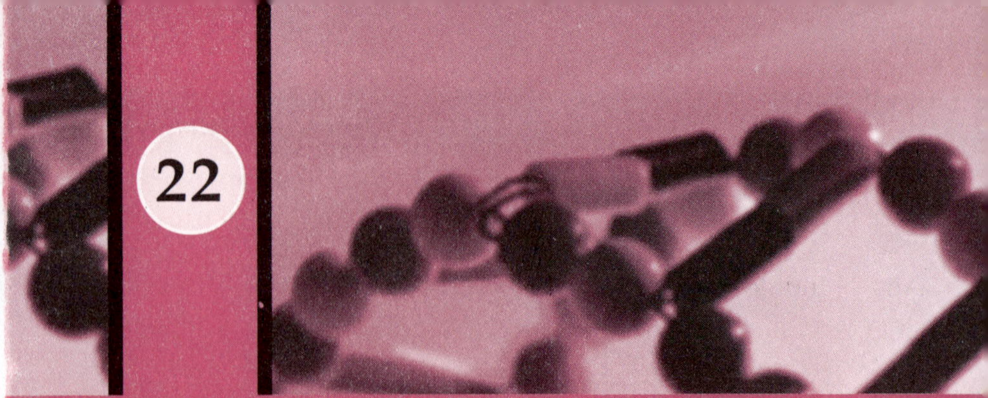

22

Biophysics

Q.1. What is pH?

Ans. It is defined as the negative logarithm of the hydrogen ion concentration.

$$pH = -\log [H^+] \text{ or}$$

$$pH = \log \frac{1}{H^+}$$

Q.2. What is the relationship between H^+ ion and the pH?

Ans. There is an inverse relationship between the two. As the H^+ ion concentration increases, the pH decreases and vice versa.

Q.3. What are the methods by which pH of any solution can be determined?

Ans. 1. Indicator papers

2. pH paper

3. pH meter

Q.4. What is the pH of distilled water, gastric juice, pancreatic juice, blood and urine?

Ans. 1. Distilled water : 7.0

2. Gastric juice : 1.6-1.8

3. Pancreatic juice : 8-9
4. Blood : 7.4 (7.35-7.45)
5. Urine : 4.8-8.0, average being 6.0

Q.5. What are buffers?

Ans. Buffers are solutions which resist changes in their pH when small amount of acids or alkalies are added to them. These are like shock absorbers against sudden changes of pH.

Q.6. What is the composition of a buffer?

Ans. Buffer is a pair of weak acid and its salt with a strong base.

Example: CH_3COOH/CH_3COONa

Q.7. Give few examples of commonly used buffers in the laboratory.

Ans. 1. Acetate buffer (sodium acetate/acetic acid)
2. Citrate buffer (sodium citrate/citric acid)
3. Phosphate buffer (Na_2HPO_4/KH_2PO_4)

Q.8. How the pH of a buffer solution can be calculated?

Ans. It can be calculated by Henderson-Hasselbalch equation:

$$pH = pK + \log \frac{\text{Concentration of salt}}{\text{Concentration of acid}}$$

Q.9. What is pK?

Ans. pK is that pH at which the acid is half neutralised.

Q.10. Name various buffers of blood.

Ans. 1. CO_2/HCO_3^-
2. $H.Hb/Hb^-$
3. $H.HbO_2/HbO_2^-$
4. H. Protein/Protein$^-$
5. $H_2PO_4^-/HPO_4^{--}$

Q.11. Name the various buffers of CSF and ECF.

Ans. 1. CO_2/HCO_3^-
2. H. Protein/Protein$^-$
3. H_2PO_4/HPO_4^{--}

Q.12. Name the important cations of the body/body fluids.

Ans. Na^+, K^+, Ca^{++} etc.

Q.13. Name the important anions of the blood/body fluids.

Ans. Bicarbonate (HCO_3^-), Chloride (Cl^-), Phosphate (HPO_4) etc.

Q.14. What do you understand by pH scale?

Ans. 1. Neutral pH 7.0
2. Acidic pH 0 - 6.9
3. Alkaline pH 7.0 - 14

Q.15. What do you understand by emulsion?

Ans. 1. They are liquid/liquid colloids
2. The two liquids are immiscible
3. Either liquid can be dispersed in the other

Q.16. What is the commonest example of emulsion?

Ans. Milk is the commonest example which contains droplets of liquid fat dispersed in an aqueous medium. The emulsifier is the protein called ***casein.***

Q.17. Who is the father of colloidal chemistry?

Ans. Graham.

Q.18. Define colloids. Give examples.

Ans. Substances which do not pass through the parchment paper while in solution are called as colloids (glue-like). Examples are albumin, gelatin etc.

Q.19. What is the physiological importance of colloids?

Ans. 1. Enzyme action
2. Maintenance of blood pH
3. Fat absorption and protection of bile contents
4. Water transport
5. Formation of urine
6. Donnan membrane equilibrium

Q.20. What is dialysis?

Ans. The retention of colloidal particles by a parchment membrane and passage of dispersion medium is called dialysis. This is employed to filter off the colloidal particles.

Q.21. What is osmosis?

Ans. It is defined as the spontaneous flow of water into a solution or from a more dilute to a more concentrated solution when the two solutions are separated from each other by a semi-permeable membrane. Osmosis occurs in the direction opposite to that in which diffusion occurs.

Q.22. What is osmotic pressure?

Ans. It is defined as the equivalent of excess pressure which must be applied to the solution to prevent the passage of the solvent into it through a semi-permeable membrane separating the two.

Q.23. How will you determine the viscosity of blood?

Ans. With the help of Hess Viscometer.

Q.24. How many times blood is viscous than water?

Ans. Nearly 4.5 times.

Q.25. In which clinical conditions viscosity of blood is lowered?

Ans.
1. Anaemia
2. Nephritis
3. Leukaemia
4. Malaria
5. Jaundice
6. Pneumonia
7. Diabetes mellitus, etc.

Q.26. Name the conditions in which viscosity of the blood gets increased.

Ans.
1. Excessive sweating, and
2. Traumatic shock

Q.27. Name any congenital disease in which viscosity of blood gets increased.

Ans. Waldenstrom's macroglobulinemia.

Q.28. How will you determine the pH of urine?

Ans. Either by (a) pH meter or (b) narrow range pH strips.

Q.29. Does any solution contain pH above 14?

Ans. No

Q.30. Is pH 1 more acidic or pH 6?

Ans. pH 1 is more acidic.

Q.31. Is pH 8 more alkaline or pH 13?

Ans. pH 13

Q.32. What is the pH of milk?

Ans. 7.1

Q.33. What are isotopes?

Ans. These may be defined as atoms of the same element having the same atomic number but different atomic weights.

Q.34. Give some examples of stable isotopes.

Ans.
1. ^{2}H (deuterium, heavy hydrogen)
2. ^{15}N
3. ^{18}O
4. ^{13}C

Q.35. Give some examples of radioactive isotopes (radioisotopes).

Ans.
1. ^{14}C
2. ^{32}P
3. ^{131}I
4. ^{60}CO
5. ^{3}H
6. ^{59}Fe, etc.

Q.36. Which isotopes are generally used for treatment purposes in clinical medicine?

Ans.
1. ^{131}I
2. ^{32}P, etc.

Q.37. With the help of which instrument(s), radioactive isotopes are detected?

Ans.
1. Geiger Muller counter
2. Scintillation counters

Q.38. With the help of which instrument, stable isotopes are detected?

Ans. Mass spectrograph.

Q.39. What is the property of a radioactive isotope?

Ans. It is unstable and decomposes spontaneously emitting out α, β or γ radiations.

Q.40. What is half life?

Ans. It is the time taken for the disappearance of half of its original isotope.

Q.41. What is the effect of a radioactive isotope on a human cell?

Ans. 1. It inactivates enzymes of the cell, vis-a-vis completely paralyses its functioning.
2. It causes structural changes in the chromosomes.
3. It is also responsible for various chemical changes in the genes.

Q.42. Do malignant (cancerous) cells take-up more or less of isotopes?

Ans. More, hence are readily detected.

Q.43. In which conditions radioactive iodine (^{131}I) has got medical use?

Ans. 1. Hyperthyroidism
2. Carcinoma of thyroid
3. In determining functional activity of the thyroid gland

Q.44. What are the uses of isotopes in medicine?

Ans. A. Its main uses are in the study of various metabolisms of the body, viz.:
1. Carbohydrate metabolism : ^{14}C glucose, ^{14}C acetate are used
2. Lipid metabolism : ^{14}C acetate is used
3. Protein metabolism ^{14}C and ^{15}N leucine, etc. are used.
4. Nucleoprotein metabolism: radioactive thymidine, etc. are used.

B. Besides, they are also used extensibly in enzymology for knowing active sites of enzymes like chymotrypsin and choline esterase etc.

C. Still, they are also used in the diagnosis and treatment of various diseases.

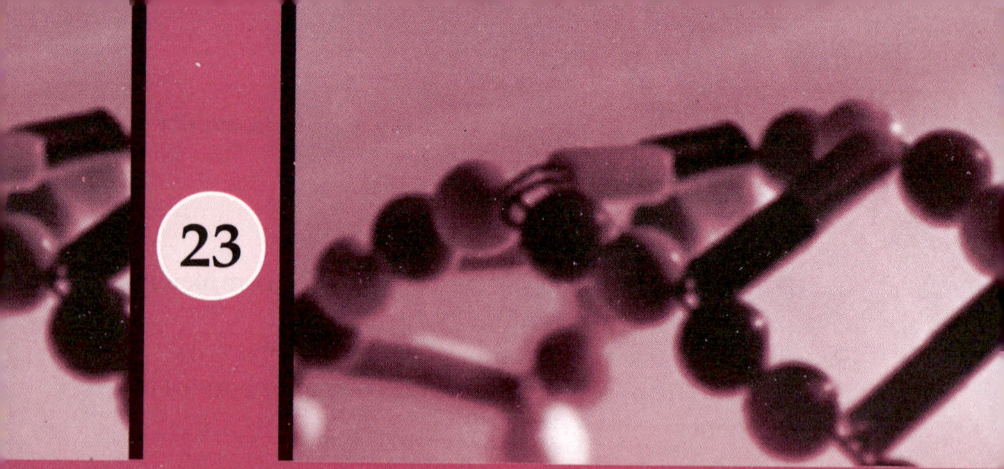

23

COLORIMETRY

Q.1. What is Lambert's law?

Ans. It states that the proportion of the light absorbed by an absorbing substance is independent of the intensity of the incident light.

Q.2. What is Beer's law?

Ans. Beer's law states that the proportion of light absorbed depends only on the total number of absorbing molecules through which light passes.

Q.3. What is optical density?

Ans. It is the logarithmic ratio of the intensity of the incident light to that of the emergent light.

$$\text{O.D.} = \log 10 \frac{I_o}{I}$$

where I_o = Intensity of incident light; I = Intensity of the emergent light.

Q.4. What is transmission?

Ans. Transmission is defined as the ratio of the intensity of the transmitted light to that of the incident light.

$$T = \frac{I_o}{I}$$

where I_o = intensity of incident light; I = intensity of the emergent light.

Q.5. What is the relation between the optical density and transmittance?

Ans. Optical density (O.D.) and transmittance are related by the formula: Optical density = 2 - log (transmittance)

Q.6. What is the use of blank in colorimetric estimations?

Ans. The function of blank is to eliminate the effect of light absorption by the reagents used, since otherwise they might lead to false high values for optical density vis-a-vis high values of the substance which is being estimated.

Q.7. What is colorimeter?

Ans. An instrument which has got the capability to measure the density of any coloured solution.

Q.8. What is the normal visible range?

Ans. 400-760 mμ

Q.9. What is photoelectric colorimetry?

Ans. When absorption measurements are done by photoelectric colorimeters in the visible region of the spectrum (i.e., between 400-760 mm of wavelength), the device is termed as photoelectric colorimetry.

Q.10. What is spectrophotometry?

Ans. If absorption measurements are done in the invisible region of spectrum (i.e., in the ultraviolet and infrared region), the technique is termed as spectrophotometry in which we make use of spectrophotometers.

Q.11. What is the normal UV range?

Ans. Less than 400 mμ.

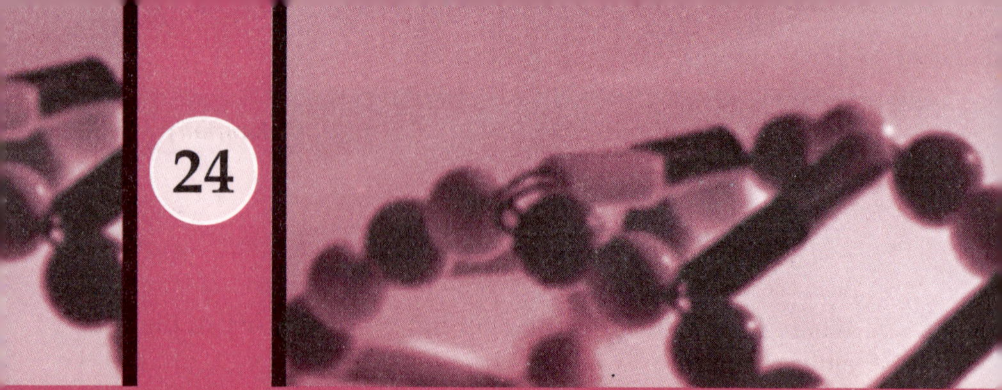

24 Miscellaneous

Q.1. How many cavities are found in the human body?

Ans. Four, namely :

(i) Cranial cavity
(ii) Thoracic cavity
(iii) Abdominal cavity, and
(iv) Pelvic cavity

Q.2. What is the composition of protoplasm?

Ans. It's composition is as follows:

(a) 60-70% water
(b) 16% proteins
(c) 14% lipids

The rest of the protoplasm is made-up of dissolved gases, inorganic salts, metals, and a small amount of carbohydrates.

Q.3. How many types of glands are there in human body?

Ans. (a) Endocrine glands, for e.g., thyroid
(b) Exocrine glands, for e.g., salivary glands

The pancreas is both endocrine and exocrine. It produces digestive enzymes that are passed to the intestine through the pancreatic duct (exocrine), but it also produces a hormone (insulin) which is transported through the body by the circulatory system (endocrine).

Q.4. Of how many vertebrae, a vertebral column is made-up of?

Ans. 26, i.e.,

(a)	**Cervical region**	:	**C_1 to C_7**
(b)	**Thoracic region**	:	**T_1 to T_{12}**
(c)	**Lumbar region**	:	**L_1 to L_5**
(d)	**Sacral region**	:	**Sacrum 1**
(e)	**Coccygeal region**	:	**Cociyx 1**

Q.5. Of how many bones skull is composed of?

Ans. 21 separate bones which remain joined together and therefore move as a unit, plus one freely movable bone, the mandible.

Q.6. What is epilepsy?

Ans. Epilepsy, once popularly called "fathing sickness" is a disease of the central nervous system (CNS) characterized by recurring convulsions and loss of consciousness that may be brief or prolonged. In most of the cases, the cause of the disorder is not known. Severe seizures are termed **'grand mal',** if the patient suffers no more than brief periods of dizziness or loss of memory.

Q.7. What do you mean by osteoporosis?

Ans. Porus bones.

Q.8. Is the estimation of homocysteine in blood a marker of the functioning of various diseases/organs?

Ans. While **high levels** of homocysteine in blood (hyperhomocysteinemia) have been found to be associated with cardiovascular, renal diseases, etc. There are reports of its **low levels** (hypohomocysteinemia) in **pregnancy.**

Q.9. What is metastasis?

Ans. It is the spread of cells to other organs.

Q.10. What is the definition of basal metabolic rate (BMR)?

Ans. It is the amount of energy expanded by the body to maintain its vital functions when it is at rest.

Q.11. By the deficiency of which enzyme, thiamine deficiency is detected?

Ans. **Transketolase** in blood.

Q.12. In which disease/condition, activity of transketolase enzyme gets elevated in blood?

Ans. Pernicious anaemia.

Q.13. What is chylothorax?

Ans. In chylothorax, there is an abnormal connection between the pleural space and the lymphatic drainage of the small intestine that results in the accumulation of **milky pleural fluid;** in this disorder production of **chyle** gets increased.

Q.14. How will you calculate LDL-cholesterol if you know the values of total and HDL cholesterol & TG in blood?

Ans. LDL cholesterol = Total cholesterol - (HDL cholesterol - TG/5)

Q.15. What are the main biochemical functions of omega-3 (OMG-3) fatty acids?

Ans. They have the following important roles in the human body :

(i) They prevent the formation of unwanted blood clots by keeping the levels of **thromboxanes** in check; thus protect heart from ailments.

(ii) They also increase the **flexibility of the red blood cell membranes,** enabling these cells to flow more freely through the complex network of the tiny capillaries. This, not only improves circulation, but makes it easier for the heart to pump blood constantly; **thus, protect heart from various disorders.**

(iii) They are natural **blood thinners** and also keep the blood fats known as triglycerides down in acceptable range, lower blood pressure and help the arteries stay elastic and free of inflammation.

(iv) They can control the **immune system** from reeling out of control, thus increase immune system.

(v) They help prevent insulin resistance; thus, play important role in the prevention of **diabetes mellitus**.

(vi) They safeguard eyes against **glaucoma** which is caused by poor circulation in the arteries that feed the eye. This puts pressure on the optic nerves causing damage to the eye. These are natural helpers in preventing such blood disorders, thus prevent eye problems.

(vii) Intake of omega-3-fatty acids is very good in pregnancy for the growth of cells and the development of various foetal functions. Therefore, the more **OMG 3** enriched foods a pregnant woman includes in her diet, the more nourishment she provides to the unborn child. Thus, they play a good role in **healthy pregnancy.**

Q.16. An alpha helix of a protein is most likely to be disrupted if a missense mutation introduces one of the following amino acids within the α-helical structure :

(a) Alanine
(b) Aspartic acid
(c) Tyrosine
(d) Glycine

Ans. Aspartic acid.

Q.17. During gluconeogenesis, reducing equivalents are transported from mitochondria to cytosol by any one of the following :

(a) Aspartate
(b) Oxaloacetate
(c) Malate
(d) Glutamate

Ans. Malate.

Q.18. What is glucagonoma?

Ans. The α-cell islet tumours of the pancreas are mostly malignant and demonstrate progressive metastatic growth. The diagnosis is established by the appearance of clinical symptoms and by the finding of a **plasma glucagon level exceeding 500 ng/l.**

Q.19. The following separation technique depends upon the molecular size of the protein :

(a) Chromatography on a carboxymethyl (CM) cellulose column

(b) Iso-electric focussing
(c) Gel filtration chromatography
(d) Chromatography on a diethylaminoethyl (DEAE) cellulose column.

Ans. Gel filtration chromatography.

Q.20. At physiological pH, the DNA molecules are :
(a) Positively charged
(b) Negatively charged
(c) Amphipathic
(d) Neutral

Ans. Negatively charged and amphipathic.

Q.21. One of the following hormones does not have any intracellular receptor :
(a) Vitamin D_3
(b) Cortisone
(c) Adrenaline
(d) Thyroxine

Ans. Adrenaline

Q.22. Accumulation of sphingomyelin in phagocytes is a feature of :
(a) Gaucher's disease
(b) Niemann–Pick disease
(c) Tay–Sach's disease
(d) Down syndrome

Ans. Niemann-Pick disease

Q.23. Accumulation of GM_2 gangliosides is a feature of :
(a) Gaucher's disease
(b) Niemann–Pick disease
(c) Tay-Sach's disease
(d) Down syndrome

Ans. Tay-Sach's disease

Q.24. Accumulation of glucosyl ceramide is a feature of :
(a) Gaucher's disease
(b) Niemann–Pick disease
(c) Tay-Sach's disease
(d) Down syndrome

Ans. Gaucher's disease

Q.25. In hemoglobin, the innate affinity of heme for CO is diminished by the presence of :

- **(a) His F-8**
- **(b) His E-7**
- **(c) Gly B-6**
- **(d) Thr C-4**

Ans. His E-7

Q.26. Name the most important signalling substance of the human brain and the nervous system.

Ans. Acetylcholine

Q.27. Name the first Japanese to be awarded Nobel Prize for Physiology or Medicine and in which year?

Ans. Tonegawa, Susumu (1987).

Q.28. What was the field of first Nobel Laureate of Japan for Physiology or Medicine?

Ans. Immunological studies (antibodies)

Q.29. Who is the father of modern chemotherapy?

Ans. **Paul Ehrlich (contribution to Immunology)**. He was the founder and first Director of what is now known as the **Paul Ehrlich Institute.**

Q.30. In which year father of modern chemotherapy was awarded Nobel Prize?

Ans. 1908

Q.31. Who discovered antibiotic 'penicillin'?

Ans. Sir Alexander Fleming in 1928.

Q.32. Name the fungus from which 'penicillin' is produced.

Ans. Penicillium notatum

Q.33. In which year, Fleming was awarded Nobel Prize?

Ans. 1945

Q.34. Most direct precursor of taurine is:

- **(a) Glycine**
- **(b) Cysteine**
- **(c) Methionine**
- **(d) Glutathione**

Ans. (b) Cysteine

Q.35. The most important buffer in RBCs is:

(a) O_2. Hb + Na Hemoglobinate
(b) O_2. Hb + K Hemoglobinate
(c) $H_2\ CO_3$ + K HCO_3
(d) $H_2\ CO_3$ + Na HCO_3

Ans. (b) O_2. Hb + K Hemoglobinate

Q.36. Iron in hemoglobin is held by :

(a) Polar bonds
(b) Non-polar bonds
(c) Co-ordinate bonds
(d) Covalent bonds

Ans. (c) Co-ordinate bonds

Q.37. Rigor Mortis is known as :

(a) Relaxation of muscles
(b) Loss of NAD
(c) Deficiency of enzyme hexokinase
(d) Deficiency of enzyme PFK
(e) None

Ans. (e) None

Q.38. Muscle relaxation means:

(a) More production of ATP
(b) More production of CTP
(c) Dissociation of actin and myosin and a decrease in the cross-linking between these elements.
(d) The loss of high energy reserve i.e. creatine PO_4 in muscles.

Ans. (c) Dissociation of actin and myosin and a decrease in the cross-linking between these elements.

Q.39. What is Rigor Mortis?

Ans. **Rigor Mortis** is the stiffening of muscles that occurs after death which is associated with the fall in ATP level as the rate of breakdown of ATP by muscle ATPase exceeds the rate of ATP synthesis.

The signs of **rigor mortis** appear when the ATP level falls to 85 percent of its initial value, and it is practically complete when the ATP level has touched 15 percent of this value. It appears that factors other than decreased

ATP levels may be involved in rigor, but these are imperfectly understood.

In nutshell, **Rigor Mortis is stiffening of muscles due to depletion of ATP reserves in the muscles.**

Q.40. What is HIV?

Ans. HIV is human immuno-deficiency virus

Q.41. What is AIDS?

Ans. AIDS is Acquired, Immunodeficiency Syndrome

Q.42. What type of disease is HIV?

Ans. It is a viral disease which knocks out the immune system and makes the person vulnerable to infectious diseases. AIDS is the late stage of infection leading to death.

Q.43. How is HIV transmitted?

Ans. It is transmitted through :

(i) Semen and vaginal fluids
(ii) Receiving infected blood and blood products
(iii) Infected pregnant mother to her baby during birth
(iv) Breast milk
(v) Contaminated needles

Q.44. How to avoid HIV infection?

Ans. By responsible sexual behaviour only i.e.

(i) Avoiding multiple sex partners
(ii) Use of condoms
(iii) Use of tested blood free of HIV
(iv) Use of clean sterilized/disposable syringes and needles.
(v) Timely treatment of sexually transmitted diseases

Q.45. HIV is not spread by:

Ans. (i) Shaking hands with a positive person
(ii) Eating together or sharing a spoon or tumbler with a positive person
(iii) Not spread by insects
(iv) Hugging or kissing a positive person
(v) Working together with an infected person
(vi) Mere skin contact or through clothes/towels etc. of a positive person

(vii) Sharing a swimming pool with HIV positive persons.

Q.46. How is diagnosis of HIV done?

Ans. (i) HIV infection is diagnosed on the basis of blood tests using three different ELISA/Rapid, simple tests using different antigen preparations.

(ii) AIDS cases are diagnosed on the basis of two different ELISA/Rapid tests on different antigens and presence of AIDS related opportunistic infections.

(iii) **Western Blot test is used for confirmation of diagnosis of indeterminate ELISA tests.**

Q.47. What is the treatment of AIDS at present?

Ans. Presently there is no cure for AIDS.

Q.48. What are steroids? Are they harmful or helpful to the human body?

Ans. Steroids are a class of structurally related, fat soluble organic compounds based on a system of 17 carbon-atom and hydrogen rings. They are widely distributed in animal and plant cells. Included in the steroid family are sterols (a group of predominantly unsaturated solid alcohols such as cholesterol and ergosterol which are found in the fatty tissues of animals and plants), vitamin-D, sex hormones, bile acids and cortisones. **The last mentioned are used in the treatment of asthma, rheumatic fever and other diseases.**

Steroids also include naturally occurring drugs such as digitalis compounds. **Some steroids are misused for artificially enhancing sporting performance and muscle building, but these have been banned.**

Steroids can, thus, be both helpful and harmful to the human body depending upon as to how they are being used.

Q.49. Who is the Architect and Father of Modern Indian Poultry Industry?

Ans. Padamshri Dr. B.V. Rao.

Q.50. What is the action of flavonoids?

Ans. Flavonoids prevent the formation of clots in the arteries and also responsible for proper circulation of blood in the arteries.

Q.51. Give the correct answer (s).

Sarcoplasm contains large store of :

(a) Glucose

(b) Fructose

(c) Maltose

(d) Glycogen

(e) Galactose

Ans. Glycogen

Q.52. Give the correct answer (s)

The phenothiazines are widely used as :

(a) Antitubercular drug

(b) Anticancer drug

(c) Antipsychotic drug

(d) Antidiabetic drug

(e) Antihelminthitic drug

Ans. Antipsychotic drug

Q.53. In cardiac muscle, the extracellular fluid is a major source of .... for excitation.

Ans. Ca^{++}

Q.54. Pteroylglutamic acid appears to be specific in the treatment of .... anaemia of pregnancy.

Ans. Megaloblastic

Q.55. Aminopterin and its derivatives, especially 10-methyl aminopterin and .... are used in the treatment of leukaemia, lymphoblastoma and trophoblastic tumors.

Ans. Methotrexate

Q.56. Antimalarial compound .... which contains in it a 2, 4 – diamino heterocyclic ring, can also combine firmly with dihydrofolic reductase and thus is a folic acid antagonist.

Ans. Pyrimethamine

Q.57. **Increase in serotonin concentration stimulates the central nervous system, an action which has been exploited in the treatment of mental depression by the administration of drugs which inhibit .... enzyme activity.**

Ans. Monoamine oxidase

Q.58. **From which amino acid, biosynthesis of epinephrine (adrenaline) and norepinephrine (nor-adrenaline) takes place?**

Ans. Tyrosine

Q.59. **Name the structural and functional unit of life.**

Ans. Cell

Q.60. **Which element is found abundantly in biomolecules?**

Ans. Carbon

Q.61. **Name the subcellular organelle where hydrolytic enzymes of the cell remain localized.**

Ans. lysosomes.

Q.62. **Who has been awarded 2016 Nobel Prize for medicine or Physiology and what is his/her field?**

Ans. Yoshinori Ohshumi (Japanese Cell Biologist) for his work on 'autophagy' (self-eating).

Q.63. **Name the pigment that gets deposited in the cells as the age advances.**

Ans. Lipofuscin.

Q.64. **Where the enzymes of energy metabolism remain present in prokaryotic cell?**

Ans. Cell membrane

Q.65. **Name any two scavengers of free radicals.**

Ans. Vitamin E and Selegiline (MAO inhibitor)

Q.66. **Name the pigment responsible for aging.**

Ans. Lipofuscin

Q.67. **1000 ml is equivalent to how much 'c.c.'?**

Ans. 1000.027 c.c.

Q.68. **What are the atomic weights of carbon, calcium, chlorine, gold, iodine, nitrogen, potassium, Na, sulphur and silver?**

Ans. 12, 40, 35.5, 197, 127, 14, 39, 23, 32 and 108 respectively.

Q.69. What are the boiling points of acetone, chloroform, CCl_4, ethanol, and toluene respectively?

Ans. 56.5°C, 61°C, 78°C, 78°C, 111°C respectively.

Q.70. Name the commonest site of melanotic tumour.

Ans. Eye

Q.71. What is the length and thickness of uterus?

Ans. About 3 inches long and 3 inches thick.

Q.72. During pregnancy, how many times uterus can increase in size?

Ans. About 20 times.

Q.73. Name the scientists who have won the Nobel Prize twice.

Ans. (1) Marie Curie,
(2) John Berdeen,
(3) Frederick Sanger, and
(4) Linus Carl Pauling

Q.74. Who has been awarded 2016 Nobel Prize for Physiology or Medicine and what is his/her field?

Ans. **Yoshinori Ohshumi** (Japanese Cell Biologist) for his work on **'autophagy' (self-eating).**

Q.75. Which sugar is the energy source of sperms?

Ans. Fructose

Q.76. Who discovered that, fructose is the energy source of sperms?

Ans. Scientist Thaddeus Mann in the year 1945

Q.77. What is the requirement of temperature for normal sperm production?

Ans. It's about 2-3°C below core body temperature

Q.78. What is the sperm range when one is called as infertile?

Ans. Less than 20 millions/ml

Q.79. What is the pH of semen?

Ans. 7.2-7.7

APPENDICES

- **Appendix-I :** Rate limiting steps (enzymes) of various Metabolic Pathways
- **Appendix-II :** Glycemic Index (GI) of Common Fruits and Vegetables
- **Appendix-III :** Biochemical Values in Blood/Plasma/Serum
- **Appendix-IV :** Desired Lipid Profile
- **Appendix-V :** Important Tumor Markers
- **Appendix-VI :** Commonly Used Anticoagulants
- **Appendix-VII :** Plasma and Urine abnormalities encountered in diseases

APPENDIX-I

Rate limiting steps (enzymes) of various Metabolic Pathways

Sl.	Pathway	Rate limiting step (enzyme)
1.	de novo pyrimidine synthesis	Aspartate transcarbamoylase (ATCase)
2.	de novo purine synthesis	Glutamine-PRPP amidotransferase
3.	Glycolysis	Phosphofructokinase-1 (PFK-1)
4.	Gluconeogenesis	Fructose-1, 6-bisphosphatase (F-1, 6-BPase)
5.	TCA cycle	Isocitrate dehydrogenase (ICDH)
6.	Glycogenesis	Glycogen synthase
7.	Glycogenolysis	Glycogen phosphorylase
8.	HMP shunt	Glucose-6-phosphate dehydro-genase (G6PD)
9.	Fatty acid synthesis	Acetyl-CoA carboxylase (ACC) (uses citrate shuttle)
10.	Fatty acid oxidation	Carnitine acyltransferase (uses carnitine shuttle)
11.	Ketogenesis	HMG-CoA synthase
12.	Cholesterol synthesis	HMG-CoA reductase (inhibited by statins)
13.	Heme synthesis	ALA synthase
14.	Urea cycle	Carbamoyl phosphate synthase I
15.	Bile acid synthesis	7-α-hydroxylase

APPENDIX-II

Glycemic Index (GI) of Common Fruits and Vegetables

Eating healthy is important to **control diabetes.** Fruits and vegetables are important parts of a healthy diet. Knowing both the **glycemic index** as well as the glycemic load of some of the more common fruits and vegetables will help one certainly to choose the favourite to incorporate in one's diet. Manage accordingly.

FRUITS	Glycemic index (glucose=100)	Serving size (grams)	Glycemic load per serving
Apple, average	39	120	6
Banana, ripe	62	120	16
Dates, dried	42	60	18
Grape fruit	25	120	3
Grapes, average	59	120	11
Orange, average	40	120	4
Peach, average	42	120	5
Pear, average	38	120	4
Prunes, pitted	29	60	10
Raisins	64	60	28
Watermelon	72	120	4
VEGETABLES			
Green peas, average	51	80	4
Carrots, average	35	80	2
Parsnips (चुकन्दर)	52	80	4
Baked russet (reddish-brown) potato, average	111	150	33
Boiled white potato, average	82	150	21
Instant mashed potato, average	87	150	17
Sweet potato, average	70	150	22
Yam (root of a tropical plant, अरुई), average	54	150	20

- Low GI foods : Have a GI of 55 or less
- Medium GI foods : Between 56 and 69
- High GI foods : 70 or higher

Note :

1. For **glycemic load,** under 10 is considered low, 10-20 is considered medium, and over 20 is considered high.

2. **Cooking time :**

   The longer a food is cooked, the higher it tends to be on the GI. When a food is cooked, the starch or carbohydrates start to break down.

3. **Fibre content :**

   In general, foods that are rich in fibre have lower glycemic ratings. The fibrous coatings around beans and seeds mean the body breaks them down more slowly. Therefore, they tend to be lower on the glycemic scale than foods without this coating.

Process :

As a general rule, the more processed a food is, the higher it is on the glycemic scale. For example, fruit juices are on a higher GI rating than fresh fruits, therefore, canned juices should be avoided.

Ripeness :

The more ripe a fruit or vegetable, the **higher** it tends to be on the GI.

APPENDIX-III: Biochemical Values in Blood / Plasma / Serum

Sl. No.	Constituent	Normal Range	High in	Low in
DIABETES MELLITUS				
1.	(a) Blood sugar (fasting) (b) Serum glucose (SI unit)	70-100 mg/dl 4.2-6.1 mmol/l	Diabetes mellitus, hyperthyroidism, hyperadrenalism hyperpituitarism etc. (for example, Simmonds' disease).	Hyperinsulinism, hypothyroidism (myxoedema, cretinism), hypoadrenalism (Addison's disease) and hypopituitarism
	(c) Glucose (random)	80-120 mg/dl	-do-	-do-
2.	Blood sugar (P.P. i.e., after 2 hrs of 75 g glucose or routine full meal)	Less than 140 mg/dl	-do-	-do-
3.	Glycosylated or glycated haemoglobin (HbA_{1C})	(a) 4.5 - 6.0% (b) 5.7 - 6.4% (indicates increased risk of diabetes mellitus) (c) 6.5% and above (indicates D.M.)	Diabetes mellitus (upto 20%)	-
RENAL FUNCTION TESTS				
1.	(a) Blood urea (b) Blood urea (SI units) (c) Urea Nitrogen	14-43 mg/dl 2.2-7.2 mmol/l 6-20 mg/dl	Glomerulonephritis, chronic pyelonephritis, nephrotic syndromes, massive gastrointestinal hemorrhage, severe dehydration, obstruction in the urinary tract due to benign hyperplasia of the prostate, bilateral ureteral obstruction due to carcinoma or calculus in the urinary bladder.	Nephrosis

Contd

Sl. No.	Constituent	Normal Range	High in	Low in
2.	(a) Serum creatinine (b) Serum creatinine (SI units)	0.1-1.2 mg/dl 44-124 μ mol/l	Renal failure, congestive heart failure, shock and mechanical obstruction of the urinary tract.	-
LIVER FUNCTION TESTS				
1.	Serum bilirubin	0.2-1.0 mg/dl	Obstructive jaundice, hemolytic jaundice, neonatal jaundice, and hepatitis.	-
2.	Direct (conjugated) bilirubin	0.0-0.2 mg/dl	Hepatitis	-
3.	Indirect (unconjugated) bilirubin = Total bilirubin-direct i.e., conjugated bilirubin	0.2-0.8 mg/dl	Haemolytic jaundice and neonatal jaundice	-
4	(a) Serum cholesterol (total)	150-200 mg/dl (3.9-5.2 mmol/l in S.I units)	Diabetes mellitus, hypothyroidism, obstructive jaundice, cirrhosis of liver, nephrotic syndrome, atherosclerosis, etc.	Acute hepatitis, malnutrition anaemia, occasionally in hyperthyroidism and Gaucher's disease
	(b) Free cholesterol	25-30% of the total cholesterol	Xanthomatous biliary cirrhosis	-
	(c) Esterified cholesterol	70-75% of the total cholesterol,		Liver diseases, infective hepatitis, acute hepatic necrosis

Contd

Sl. No.	Constituent	Normal Range	High in	Low in
5.	GOT (AST)*; Glutamic oxaloacetic transaminase (Aspartate transaminase) **(Peak in 4-6 hrs after MI)**	8-40 units/ml or 4-17 IU/l	Myocardial infarction, liver disorders, skeletal muscle trauma or regeneration, etc.	-
6.	GPT (ALT)*; Glutamic pyruvic transaminase (Alanine transaminase)	5-35 units/ml or 3-15 IU/l	Liver disorders and the increase is significantly higher than SGOT. Determination of SGPT can be useful in showing the severity and prognosis of the disease.	-
7.	Alkaline phosphatase*	4-11 KA units or 60-160 IU/l	Diseases of the liver primarily with destructive or obstructive pathology (e.g., hepatitis, cirrhosis, chemical toxicity, gall-stones, biliary duct obstructions, and primary or metastatic or 'space occupying' lesions of the liver), bony lesions (e.g. osteogenic sarcoma, metastatic carcinomas, rickets, Paget's disease) and also with primary and secondary parathyroidism.	Scurvy, severe anemia, malnutrition, achondroplasia, cretinism, hypophosphatasia

Contd

Sl. No.	Constituent	Normal Range	High in	Low in
8	(a) Serum total proteins (b) Serum total proteins (S.I. units)	6.0-8.0 g/dl 60-80 g/l	Multiple myeloma and conditions associated with high globulin concentration.	Different clinical conditions associated with nephrotic syndromes, neoplastic disease, malnutrition, Kwashiorkor syndrome, cirrhosis of liver and other liver disorders.
9.	(a) Serum albumin (b) Serum albumin (S.I. units)	3.5-5.0 g/dl 35-50 g/l	Pathological conditions associated with increased levels of serum albumin are not known.	Different conditions such as cirrhosis of liver, other liver disorders, nephrotic syndromes, malnutrition, malignancies, chronic protracted conditions like ulcerative colitis.
10.	Serum globulins	2.3-3.6 g/dl	Advanced liver diseases	-
11.	Fibrinogen (plasma)	0.3-0.6 g/dl	Infections	Cirrhosis of liver, acute hepatic necrosis, poisoning by carbon tetrachloride, etc.
12.	Albumin/Globulins ratio (ratio gets reversed in advanced liver diseases)	1.2-1.5	-	Less than 1 in liver diseases and high in chronic infections
13.	Gamma glutamyl transferase (γ-GT)*	11-50 IU/l (men) 7 -32 IU/l (women)	Biliary obstruction and alcoholism	

Contd

Sl. No.	Constituent	Normal Range	High in	Low in
PANCREATIC FUNCTION TESTS				
1.	Amylase*	80-180 Somogyi units	Pancreatitis, stone and cancer in biliary duct	
2.	Serum lipase	Less than 150 U/l	Pancreatitis, cancer in pancreas, cirrhosis, hepatitis, duodenal ulcer, diseases of the biliary tract, etc.	
LIPID PROFILE				
1.	(a) Serum cholesterol (total)	150-200 mg/dl (3.9-5.2 mmol/l in S.I. units)	Diabetes mellitus, hypothyroidism, obstructive jaundice, cirrhosis of liver, nephrotic syndrome, atherosclerosis, etc.	Acute hepatitis, malnutrition anaemia, occasionally in hyperthyroidism and Gaucher's disease
	(b) HDL cholesterol	30-63 mg/dl (men) 35-75 mg/dl (women)	The combined risk factor of coronary heart disease (CHD) can be determined following the estimations of serum cholesterol and HDL - cholesterol	-
	(c) LDL - cholesterol**	40 - 130 mg/dl	The ratio of cholesterol to HDL cholesterol has predictive value in determining the risk of CHD more accurately. **For normal males the ratio of 5:1 and for normal females the ratio of 4.5:1 are considered as average risk.** Lower ratios significantly	-

Contd

Sl. No.	Constituent	Normal Range	High in	Low in
			reduce the risk, whereas ratios 9.5:1 and 7:1 for males and females respectively, are believed to double the risk of CHD. An inverse relationship has been observed between the risk of CHD and the concentration of HDL - cholesterol. HDL cholesterol represents approximately 20-25% of the total cholesterol in serum.	
	(d) VLDL	upto 28 mg/dl	Hyperlipidemia	-
	(e) Lipoprotein 'a' i.e., Lp (a)	0-30 mg/dl	Atherosclerosis, heart attack or stroke	-
	(f) Free cholesterol	25-30% of the total cholesterol	Xanthomatous biliary cirrhosis	-
	(g) Esterified cholesterol	70-75% of the total cholesterol		Liver diseases, infective hepatitis, acute hepatic necrosis
2.	Triglycerides*	30-140 mg/dl	Hyperlipidemia, atherosclerosis, diabetes mellitus; nephrosis, biliary obstruction and metabolic disorders associated with certain endocrine diseases.	-

Contd

Sl. No.	Constituent	Normal Range	High in	Low in
3.	Total lipids *	360-820 mg/dl	Diabetes mellitus, biliary cirrhosis, late pregnancy, nephrosis and hypothyroidism.	Hyperthyroidism
STOMACH FUNCTION TEST				
1.	Fractional test meals (FTM) i.e., gastric analysis	Free acidity 0.0-40 meq/l Total acidity 20-55 meq/l	Duodenal ulcer and gastric ulcer	Hypochlorhydria (hypo-acidity)
ANAEMIA				
1.	(a) Haemoglobin (males) (b) Haemoglobin (females)	14-18 g/dl 11-16 g/dl	Polycythaemias, congenital Cyanotic heart disease, and in haemoconcentration due to various clinical causes e.g., heat-stroke and dehydration.	Anaemias of different kind restilting from haemorrhage or from deficiency of iron, vitamin B_{12} or folic acid. Red cell haemolysis resulting from auto-immune process or due to enzyme abnormality (G-6-PD) may result in anaemia. The defective globin chain synthesis as in thalassemias or structural abnormalities of the haemoglobin molecule as in abnormal haemoglobins may result in severe anaemia.

* in serum

Contd

** $\dfrac{\textbf{Plasma (serum) triglycerides}}{5}$ **= VLDL**

(Total serum cholesterol - HDL) - (VLDL) = LDL

Note: **Hypercholesterolaemia is known to be associated with an increased risk of coronary heart disease (CHD)**

Sl. No.	Constituent	Normal Range	High in	Low in
CARDIAC ENZYMES				
1.	GOT (AST)*; Glutamic oxaloacetic transaminase (Aspartate transaminase) **(Peak in 4-6 hrs after MI)**	8-40 units/ml or 4-17 IU/l	Myocardial infarction, liver disorders, skeletal muscle trauma or regeneration, etc.	-
2.	Serum lactic dehydrogenase (LDH) **(Peak in 8-10 hrs after MI)**	230 - 460 IU/I	Myocardial infarction, infective hepatitis, toxic jaundice, etc.	-
3.	Serum creatine phosphokinase (CPK or CK) **(Peak in 24-36 hrs after MI)**	20-50 IU/l (men) 10-37 IU/l (women)	Myocardial infarction and progressive muscular dystrophy of Duchenne type. In MI, CPK is increased earlier than GOT and LDH, beginning within 6 hrs, and at peak on an average at 24 hrs. and returning to the normal within 2-3 days. Increased levels may also be found in polymyositis and other muscular dystrophies, etc.	-
CARDIAC MARKERS				
1.	Troponin - T (c Tn T)	0 - 0.1 mg/L	Myocardial Infarction	-
2.	Troponin - I (c Tn I)		Myocardial Infarction	

Contd

Sl. No.	Constituent	Normal Range	High in	Low in
3.	Homocysteine	4.0 -12 mmol/L	Myocardial Infarction	Pregnancy
4.	Myoglobin	19-92 mg/L (M) 12-76 mg/L (F)	Myocardial Infarction (a relatively early marker, elevation after 4-6 hrs of AMI)	
THYROID FUNCTION TESTS				
1.	Triiodothyronine (T_3)	60 - 190 ng/dl (RIA method)	Pregnancy, Hyperthyroidism	Hypothyroidism
2.	Thyroxine (T_4)	1.5 - 4.0 ng/dl (RIA method)	Hyperthyroidism	Hypothyroidism
3.	TSH	0.3 - 6.0 mU/ml	Hypothyroidism	Hyperthyroidism
4.	Thyroid Binding Globulin (TBG)	2.0 - 4.8 ng/dl	Pregnancy, Acute Liver Disease Thyrotoxicosis	Major illness Nephrosis
5.	Protein Bound Iodine (PBI)	4 - 8 mg/dl	Hyperthyroidism Nephrosis, etc.	Hypothyroidism
HORMONES				
1.	Insulin	5 - 20 mU/ml (Adult Fasting)	Hypoglycemia, Insulinoma	Diabetes Mellitus
2.	Testosterone	350-1000 ng/dl , (Males) - 20 - 70 ng/dl, (Females)	Hypogonadism Elevated (females)-Adrenal or Ovarian Tumors	(Males) -

Contd

Sl. No.	Constituent	Normal Range	High in	Low in
3.	Thyrocalcitonin	20 - 400 pg/ml	Medullary carcinoma of the thyroid	-
4.	Human Chorionic Gonadotropin (HCG)	2,000-40,000 IU/l	Detectable level confirms pregnancy	Threatened pregnancy
5.	**Gastrin**	< 300 pg/ml	**Stomach or Duodenal Ulcer, Zollinger Ellison Syndrome**	-
MISCELLANEOUS				
1.	Ketone bodies (blood)	upto 3 mg%	Diabetes mellitus	-
2.	(a) Acid phosphatase (Total)* (b) Acid phosphatase (Prostatic)	1-0-4.0 KA units 0.0-0.8 KA units	Carcinoma of prostrate gland, Paget's disease and hyperparathyroidism	
3.	Serum uric acid	2.5-7.0 mg/dl (men) 1.5-6.0 mg/dl (women)	Gout, renal failure, uremia, leukaemia and following radiotherapy of lymphomas.	Wilson's disease, Fanconi syndrome, some cases of Acromegaly and following the usage of uricosuric drugs.
4.	(a) Serum calcium (b) Serum calcium (S.I. units)	9 - 11 mg/dl 2.1-2.6 mmol/l	Hyperparathyroidism, hypervitaminosis-D and associated with increased levels of thyrocalcitonin.	Tetany, hypoparathyroidism, rickets, osteomalacia, etc.

Contd

Sl. No.	Constituent	Normal Range	High in	Low in
5.	(a) Inorganic phosphorus (Adults)* (b) Inorganic phosphorus* (Children)	2.5-4.8 mg/dl (0.8-1.6 mmol/l) 4.0-7.0 mg/dl (1.3-2.3 mmol/l)	Hypoparathyroidism, renal failure, hypervitaminosis-D, etc	Rickets, hyperparathyroidism, Fanconi syndrome, etc.
6.	Renal threshold value for glucose	160-180 mg/dl	-	-
7.	Magnesium*	1-3 mg/dl	-	Vomiting and diarrhoea
8.	Lithium*	Absent or in traces	-	-
9.	Sodium*	137-148 meq/l	-	Diabetic acidosis
10.	Potassium*	3.6-5.4 meq/l	Pneumonia, acute infections and uremia.	

APPENDIX-IV : Desired Lipid Profile

Categories	Total Cholesterol mg/dl	HDL Cholesterol mg/dl	LDL Cholesterol mg/dl	VLDL mg/dl	Triglycerides mg/dl
Normal	150 - 200 (Preferably < 180)	30 - 63 (males) 35 - 75 (females)	40 - 130	28	30 - 140
Borderline high	200 - 240	...	130 - 160		140 - 200
Worrisome	more than 240	< 35	more than 160		more than 200

APPENDIX-V : Important Tumor Markers

Sl. No.	TUMOR MARKERS	ASSOCIATED CANCER
1.	Carcino Embryonic Antigen (CEA)	Colon, Lung, Breast, Pancreas
2.	Alpha Fetoprotein (AFP)	Germ cell cancers of ovaries & testes, some primary liver cancers (hepatocellular)
3.	Prostate - Specific Antigen (PSA)	Prostate Cancer
4.	Prostatic - Acid Phosphatase (PAP)	Prostate Cancer
5.	Lactic Dehydrogenase (LDH)	Lymphoma, Melanoma, Acute Leukemia
6.	Calcitonin (CT)	Medullary Cancer of the Thyroid
7.	Human Chorionic Gonadotropin (HCG)	Trophoblast i.e., neoplasia, Gonadal Germ Cell Tumor
8.	Thyroglobulin (Tg)	Thyroid Cancer
9.	Vanillylmandelic acid (VMA)	Neuroblastoma & Pheochromocytoma, Ganglioneuroma
10.	Homovanillic acid (HVA)	Neuroblastoma
11.	Bence Jones Protein	Multiple myeloma, Chronic lymphocytic leukemia (CLL)
12.	CA 125 Cancer Antigen 125 or Carbohydrate antigen 125	Ovarian cancer, breast, colorectal, uterine, cervical, pancreas, liver, lung, etc.

APPENDIX-VI : Commonly Used Anticoagulants

S.No.	Anticoagulant	mg /ml Blood	Use	Mode of Action
1.	Heparin	0. 2	Procedures requiring whole blood or plasma especially useful when intact erythrocytes are desired	Inhibits conversion of prothrombin to thrombin
2.	Ethylenediamine - tetraacetic acid (EDTA)	1	Procedures requiring whole blood or plasma	Chelates ionic calcium
3.	Oxalates (a) Lithium (b) Sodium (c) Potassium (d) Ammonium	1 - 2	Procedures requiring whole blood or plasma. Causes shrinkage of cell volume, should not be used in haematological procedures.	Forms unionized calcium oxalate complex; reduces level of ionized calcium below that required for clotting

Contd

S.No.	Anticoagulant	mg /ml Blood	Use	Mode of Action
4.	Sodium Citrate	5	As for oxalates	Forms unionized complex with calcium
5.	Sodium Fluoride	10	**Combination anticoagulant and preservative for blood glucose determination by inhibiting blood enzymes causing glycolysis;** causes erythrocyte shrinkage. Combined with thymol **(1mg +10 mg NaF)** for effective control of microbial growth in stored blood samples.	Forms unionized calcium fluoride complex

APPENDIX VII : Plasma and Urine abnormalities encountered in Diseases

S.No.	Disease	Raised amino acid (s) in Plasma	Raised amino acid (s) in Urine
1.	Phenylketonuria **(PKU)**	Phenylalanine	Phenylalanine; urine screening tests are probably positive
2.	Homocystinuria	Methionine	Methionine and homocystine
3.	Maple Syrup Urine Disease **(MSU)**	Leucine, isoleucine and valine	Leucine, isoleucine and valine, may be generalized aminoaciduria
4.	Tyrosinosis	Tyrosine, with added general aminoacidaemia if liver damage present.	General raised aminoaciduria
5.	Disorders of Urea Cycle	Citrulline, lysine, glutamine, arginine, ornithine.	As plasma and also arginosuccinic acid.

Contd

S.No.	Disease	Raised amino acid (s) in Plasma	Raised amino acid (s) in Urine
6.	Aminoaciduria	Proline and/or hydroxyproline	Proline, hydroxyproline and glycine
7.	Cystinuria	Normal	Cystine, also usually lysine, ornithine and arginine
8.	Wilson's Disease	Normal or general slight elevation	Generalized
9.	Hartnup Disease	Normal	All monocarboxylic-monoamino acids except glycine
10.	Galactosaemia	General aminoacidaemia, if liver damage. Raised plasma galactose on milk diet	General aminoaciduria and strong reaction for reducing substances